M. Pescatori
C.I. Bartram
A.P. Zbar

Clinical Ultrasound in Benign Proctology

2-D and 3-D Anal, Vaginal and Transperineal Techniques

Foreword by R.J. Nicholls

Springer

EDITORS

Mario Pescatori
Villa Flaminia Hospital
Rome, Italy

Clive I. Bartram
St. Mark's Hospital
Harrow, United Kingdom

Andrew P. Zbar
School of Clinical Medicine and Research
The University of West Indies
Queen Elizabeth Hospital, Barbados

CONTRIBUTORS

Paola De Nardi
Department of Surgery
San Raffaele Scientific Institute
Milan, Italy

Carlo Ratto
Department of Surgical Sciences
Gemelli Hospital
Rome, Italy

Maria Spyrou
Villa Flaminia Hospital
Rome, Italy

Stella Ayabaca
Villa Flaminia Hospital
Rome, Italy

Library of Congress Control Number: 2006923047

ISBN-10 88-470-0366-0 Springer Milan Berlin Heidelberg New York
ISBN-13 978-88-470-0366-8 Springer Milan Berlin Heidelberg New York

Springer is a part of Springer Science+Business Media
springer.com

Printed in Italy

Cover design: estudio Calamar, Barcelona, Spain
Typesetting: Graficando, Milan, Italy
Printing: Arti Grafiche Nidasio, Assago (MI), Italy

Foreword

A large proportion of the proctologist's work includes common benign disorders of the sphincter and pelvic floor musculature and anorectal sepsis. Ultrasound has been part of the pretreatment assessment of these for many years. It adds to clinical examination and may supply the essential information on which the management decision is taken. Most importantly it gives an objective picture of the pathology, which is vital for discussion among clinicians and radiologists as part of the decision-taking process. Thus it supplies a permanent record not only useful for diagnosis and treatment but also for assessing outcomes after treatment. It may have special medicolegal value. The role of ultrasound in research has been considerable. For example, it has enabled a greater understanding of the anatomy of the sphincter and pelvic floor and it has made a major contribution to the assessment of incontinence and its management. It can give important information beyond the clinical examination in establishing the surgical anatomy of anorectal sepsis.

Ultrasonography has developed immensely during the last twenty years. In proctology, its initial application to rectal cancer has expanded owing to the invention of probes suitable for anal and pelvic floor imaging. The introduction of three-dimensional ultrasound and, latterly, transperineal sonography has increased the opportunities and sensitivity for static and now dynamic assessment.

This book is written by authors who have played a major part in the development of ultrasonography in proctology. Therefore, it carries the authority of understanding and experience. In dealing with all aspects of benign anal and pelvic disorders, the authors give an up-to-date account of its present role with indications of potential future developments. The text is detailed and is a mine of information that will be useful to all practitioners dealing with proctological conditions. It will therefore appeal not only to surgeons and radiologists but also to gastroenterologists and primary care physicians whether in established independent practice or in training. The bibliography is extensive and will be a most valuable resource to the reader. It is clearly written and the illustrations are of high quality and very informative.

Clinical Ultrasound in Benign Proctology will be of great value to all practitioners involved in coloproctology.

March, 2006

R.J. Nicholls
Harrow, UK

Preface

Since the introduction of endoluminal ultrasound for the assessment of anorectal diseases in 1989 by Law and Bartram, the fundamental investigative algorithm for functional disorders, in particular, the management of fecal incontinence, has changed dramatically. This period of investigative ultrasonography, driven by radiologists throughout Europe and North America has changed our understanding and perspective of anorectal anatomy. It has also enabled the marriage of our knowledge of healthy and disordered anorectal physiology with the relevant imaging and has allowed surgical treatments and reconstructions to be directed using an advanced morphological interpretation. This approach has guided a sophisticated management of medical and surgical therapies towards complicated cryptogenic and inflammatory bowel disease-related perirectal sepsis, preventing recurrence and preserving continence. In the area of evacuatory dysfunction presenting to specialized pelvic floor clinics, endoanal, transperineal and transintroital ultrasound has significantly contributed to the anatomic understanding and clinical significance of rectoceles, enteroceles, rectoanal intussusception and incipient rectal prolapse, providing clinical correlates for more directed operative therapies or audiovisual-based biofeedback treatments. The recent introduction of 3-dimensional reconstructive axial ultrasound has provided a more 'surgical' view of complicated fistula-in-ano which has correlated with more expensive and less available gold standard modalities such as enhanced magnetic resonance (MR) fistulography, resulting in a specialized approach towards this problem as well as delivering a better basis for medical therapies such as fibrin glue instillation or, in specialized circumstances, anti-TNF treatments in perianal Crohn's disease. Three-dimensional ultrasound has also provided a coronal interpretation for incomplete sphincteroplasty in patients with persistent or recurrent fecal incontinence who present with suboptimal outcomes. It has also directed specialist coloproctological reoperation for those patients with objective prognostic indicators more likely to result in operative success. The recent introduction of simple transperineal sonography (although its interpretation is more involved) has created an opportunity in certain anorectal disorders to overcome some of the problems inherent to the endoluminal approach where it may have a place in those patients with endoanal luminal distortion preventing the deployment of a probe assembly. Here too, in complex perirectal infections transperineal sonography can overcome the limited focal distance of the endoanal probe in defining laterally disposed extrasphincteric fistulae as well as demonstrating translevator extensions above the puborectalis floor where coupling of an endoanal probe is relatively poor. In this circumstance, transperineal sonography can also assist in delineating whether supralevator disease is an extension of perianal infection or whether it has a primary pelvirectal origin. Comparative studies are required between these newer modalities and conventional technologies such as enhanced MR imaging, where initial data suggests that transperineal ultrasound provides complementary information rather than competitive information. The indication *par excellence* for transperineal ultrasound is the dynamic real-time interpretation of compartment interaction in patients presenting with rectal evacuation disorders where colonic transit is normal by its use of simulated defecation maneuvers and forcible straining, although there is much work required here to assess the objective effects of hysterectomy as well as the categorized interpretation of transperineal images in patients with coincident uterovaginal prolapse. What is clear is that there is an increasing onus on coloproctologists to understand, interpret and perform the range of anal ultrasonography available in patients with complex anorectal disorders and to correlate these findings with operative indications and with postoperative functional outcomes. Such a view provides stimulation for surgeons to become actively involved in the performance and accreditation of all forms of anorectal sonography. There is a need for close cooperation between radiologists and colorectal surgeons in the accreditation and training in this important modality as part of their wider colorectal apprenticeship. With this in mind, although there are several texts available discussing endoanal ultrasound, our approach here is novel, as it presents the operative techniques used based on ultrasonographic interpretations from the surgeons' point of view.

In the construction of this atlas, we are indebted to the invaluable assistance of Paola De Nardi for the coordination of the text and figures.

Mario Pescatori
Rome, Italy

Clive I. Bartram
London, United Kingdom

Andrew P. Zbar
St. Michael, Barbados

Table of Contents

1 Surgeon Performed Ultrasound in Proctological Practice: an Overview

Andrew P. Zbar

Introduction

Since endoluminal ultrasonography was first introduced in 1989 for the assessment of anal and rectal disorders by Law and Bartram, [1] it has become a staple of the coloproctological armamentarium. Following its introduction, Beynon and colleagues [2] correlated images with individual rectal and anal wall layers, (mucosa, submucosa, muscularis propria, longitudinal muscle and perirectal fat), principally for estimation of tumor infiltration of the rectum. This work was independently followed by Burnett and Bartram [3] and by Papachrysostomou et al. [4] defining the constitutive variations in normal anal anatomy with age and gender and showing a 'natural' increase in thickness of the internal anal sphincter (IAS) with advancing age.

Recently, 3-dimensional reconstruction of stacked axial images obtained with an automated puller (or incorporated into in-built probe housing) has attempted to correlate manometrically defined high-pressure zones with anatomical separations in the external anal sphincter (EAS) and with the puborectalis component of the levator ani complex [5]. This technology has also clarified the anatomical disposition of the component parts of the EAS into a 3-tiered structure, (subcutaneous, superficial and deep), which has settled a long-standing argument concerning this muscle [6] and which has been validated by endoanal magnetic resonance imaging (MRI) in the display of high-resolution coronal images [7, 8]. In addition, this technique has shown the constitutive anatomy of the longitudinal muscle [9] which has clinical relevance in the spread of perirectal sepsis [10].

Our group has extended the use of surgeon-performed ultrasonography to transperineal (transcutaneous) assessment of the perineum and pelvic floor for definition of the anterior, middle and posterior pelvic compartments in dynamic use for patients presenting with the symptom complex of evacuatory dysfunction [11, 12]. In an additional recent use, Wedemeyer and colleagues [13] and Mallouhi et al. [14] have demonstrated its clinical value in the determination of the course of complex tracks in Crohn's-related and cryptogenic perirectal sepsis respectively. Our group is currently conducting a prospective trial comparing hydrogen peroxide-enhanced endoanal ultrasonography with transperineal sonography in never operated and recurrent cryptogenic fistula-in-ano to assess the accuracy of surgeon-performed ultrasound in the determination of fistula anatomy, the delineation of the site of the internal fistula opening, the presence of significant anteroanal and retrorectal horseshoeing and the validation of Goodsall's rule in fistula orientation [15]. There has also been specific utilization of ultrasound in the pre- and postoperative assessment of patients presenting with fecal incontinence and in the follow-up of reparative sphincteroplasty [16] as well as in the determination of the tumor depth and nodal status of rectal and anal tumors to guide the selected use of curative local excision, preoperative adjuvant radiation or neoadjuvant chemoradiation [17, 18].

This review provides recommendations for surgeon-performed endoluminal and transperineal sonography in clinical proctological practice with specific clinical examples.

Ultrasound in Perianal Abscess and Fistula-in-Ano

Although the vast majority of perianal sepsis does not require specialized imaging [19], the referral practice to specialist colorectal surgeons of complex and recurrent perirectal infection dictates its use and its expert interpretation for the preoperative detection of the site of internal fistula openings and the relationship of primary and secondary tracks and abscess collections to the main sphincter muscle mass. Familiarity with the technique and technical aspects and interpretation of the images produced by hand-held ultrasonography becomes essential in a tertiary colorectal practice [20].

The indications for and type of preoperative imaging in perirectal sepsis are controversial. In those cases of cryptogenic sepsis, recurrence after surgery has been shown to be most usual when an internal fistula opening has either not been recognized or identified, as well as if there has been poor recognition of the presence and course of secondary tracks and/or abscess collections or no appreciation at the first operation of horseshoeing in either the anteroanal or retrorectal spaces [21]. It is generally recommended that specialist imaging is valuable in those cases where primary sepsis is deemed to be complex, (i.e. where a track or collection occupies more than half of the coronal length of the anorectal sphincters), when recurrence occurs unexpectedly following initial surgery by an experienced surgeon, when sepsis is thought not to be of cryptogenic origin (e.g. Crohn's disease, Behçet's syndrome or in immunodeficiency-related infection) and when there is a translevator extension or a primary extrasphincteric or suprasphincteric track as defined by Parks et al. [22]. In those cases with a translevator component, a distinction should be made between cases with a primary ischiorectal origin which have broken through the levator plate, (where ischiorectal drainage will be successful) and those patients where the origin of the sepsis is pelvirectal. In this latter circumstance, drainage of an ischiorectal collection will inevitably result in a high extrasphincteric fistula and suspicion of this pathology necessitates surface imaging with a pelvic phased-array MRI [23].

Accurate delineation of the primary track and the main puborectalis muscle will permit reoperative surgery which is sphincter sparing and which will preserve continence [24], where endoanal ultrasonography has shown a considerable accuracy compared with surgical correlation for the definition of the primary fistula track and for the delineation of the internal fistula opening [25, 26]. Comparative studies of imaging modalities have shown an overall superiority of surface MR imaging over both endoanal ultrasound [27-29] and endoluminal MR imaging probes [30, 31] and over surgery as the gold standard in the complex reoperated case. In this latter circumstance, surface MR imaging will detect collections and tracks which may go unidentified by even experienced surgeons particularly when there is attendant anal canal stenosis in the setting of the multiply reoperated case [27, 32].

More recently, hydrogen peroxide-enhancement of endoanal ultrasonography, (either pre- or intraoperatively), has resulted in an improved definition of the internal opening and of unsuspected anal fistulae and has shown intersphincteric collections which occasionally do not follow Goodsall's rule concerning the directness (or otherwise) of fistula track orientation to the anal canal [33, 34]. In this circumstance, the use of ultrasound will reduce the amount of potentially uninvolved sphincter which may be inadvertently divided if these rules are used solely as operative guidelines. Because of the destructive nature of perirectal sepsis, endoanal ultrasonography will also assist the coloproctologist in the definition of the damaging secondary effects of perirectal infection that themselves may require delayed reconstructive surgery; most notably, EAS destruction requiring delayed sphincteroplasty either separately or as part of an advancement anoplasty, IAS destruction which may benefit from an attempt at plication or augmentation, [35, 36] ano- (or recto-) vaginal fistula delineation [37] and perineal body destruction [38]. Each of these anomalies requires specialist surgical expertise and preoperative definition and the planning of their surgery will be demonstrable by dedicated surgeon-performed endoanal ultrasonongraphy. Other advantages of endoanal sonography in Crohn's-related perianal infection include its ability to objectively demonstrate transmural inflammation [39] and potentially in its response to biological modulators such as Infliximab and Thalidomide [40]. More recently, hydrogen peroxide-enhanced 3-dimensional endoanal sonographic reconstruction has proved relatively disappointing in recurrent cryptogenic cases in the delineation of secondary fistula extensions [41].

Clearly, in some circumstances, endoanal technology will not provide the level of surgical information required. Here, the course of extrasphincteric fistulae will largely not be demonstrable, nor will the likelihood of suprasphincteric fistulae and translevator extensions and in both of these settings, pelvic phased-array MR imaging will be necessary where this modality is available. The nature of ultrasonic physics is also such that a large intersphincteric abscess will create moderate acoustic impedance that may 'overcall' the collection as trans-sphincteric in nature and where such technology is largely relied upon for operative decision making, healthy sphincter may be injudiciously sacrificed. In this clinical setting, we have recently been assessing transperineal sonography using a hand-held 7.5 MHz probe (Bruel & Kjaer, Denmark) to define the course of fistula tracks and their relationship to the main puborectalis mass as well as to outline any significant horseshoeing. Preliminary evidence from Mallouhi et al. [14] using a combination of 4 and 7 MHz transducers along with colour Doppler sonography, has shown that there is a moderately high accuracy for the detection of abscess collections, the attendant hyperemia of perianal sepsis and for the correct orientation of cryptogenic fistulae, with a greater tolerance to its use in acutely painful perianal pathology than with conventional endoanal sonography.

This finding has been also suggested by Wedemeyer and colleagues using transcutaneous sonography in the assessment of patients with perianal Crohn's disease [13, 42], where an added advantage is its use when there is anal canal distortion or frank stricturing precluding the use of an endorectal probe assembly. Our preliminary experience with this transcutaneous technique suggests that it is feasible although it requires a substantial learning curve. It would appear to have an advantage in defining the course of secondary tracks and collections in the coronal plane alongside the anal canal or in the intersphincteric locale as well as the presence of significant horseshoeing and it seems to define the likelihood of an underlying fistula track in those patients with their first presentation of perirectal abscess in the absence of any external opening. It is also particularly useful in the distinction between perianal and perineal sepsis. Our initial protocol of preliminary unenhanced transperineal sonography followed by unenhanced and then enhanced endoanal sonography and finally by a last enhanced transperineal sonogram, has also shown clinical benefit in defining low anovestibular fistulae which would normally lie beyond the focal distance of endoluminal probes.

Ultrasound Assessment of Fecal Incontinence

Much of the referral practice to coloproctologists for fecal incontinence is obstetric-related, [43] where traditionally, vaginal-assisted deliveries represent the major risk factors for potentially reparable anterior EAS defects [44]. Here, damage is partly morphological and partly a result of attendant unilateral or bilateral pudendal nerve neuropathy [45] with prospective evidence to show that surgical corrective sphincteroplasty correlates with in vivo evidence of sphincter defects [46]. The true incidence of this problem is still debated with variations noted by some groups between the expected clinical number of patients presenting over prolonged follow-up in maternal clinics with post-obstetric fecal incontinence and those with asymptomatic demonstrable EAS ultrasonographic defects [47, 48].

Apart from its ability to map the EAS defect, ultrasonography may provide the surgeon with information which may be predictive for the patient regarding the longer term outcome of sphincter repair, where objective assessments of EAS atrophy [49] and the presence of coincident IAS damage, (particularly if heterogeneous), will result in suboptimal functional outcomes [35]. In this setting, it is likely that surgeon-performed sonography to assess these factors will be more directed. In clinical practice, ultrasonography guides specialist repair of EAS defects as well as redo sphincteroplasties in expert hands where the short-term outcomes are favourable if performed by experienced colorectal surgeons [50]. The greatest contributor to inadequate initial outcome is an incomplete sphincteroplasty, (particularly in the coronal extent of the defect), representing a balance between the extent of repair and excessive sphincter mobilization which has the potential to devascularize and denervate the sphincter ends. In this respect, 3-dimensional reconstructed endoanal sonongraphy has shown a correlation between the rostral extent of the EAS defect and its angle, providing some further information to the surgeon regarding the potential points of EAS weakness during surgery [51]. Recently, we have used intra- and early post-operative transperineal sonography as a guide to the adequacy of overlapping EAS repair, particularly in defining the coronal extent of the repair without the need for endoanal distraction caused by an endoluminal probe.

Surgeon-performed endosonography is of further clinical value in the definition of functional disturbances following minor anorectal surgery [52] including leakage following lateral internal anal sphincterotomy, [53] post-hemorrhoidectomy incontinence, [54] after endoanal retractor distraction [55] and following some endoanal stapling procedures [56] including the recently introduced technique of stapled hemorrhoidopexy [57].

Endoanal, Transvaginal and Dynamic Transperineal Endosonography in Functional Bowel Disorders

Dynamic transperineal ultrasonography (DTP-US) is a novel method for the real-time assessment of the anterior, middle and posterior pelvic compartments and perineal soft tissues during provocative maneuvers such as straining and simulated defecation, being utilized in patients presenting with primary evacuatory dysfunction or those with defecation difficulty following pelvic surgery [11]. There is clinically a poor correlation between the symptoms attributed to pelvic floor dysfunction and radiologically demonstrated anatomical findings, [58] where it is recognized that more than 90% of patients presenting with evacuatory difficulty to colorectal surgeons have a multiplicity of pelvic pathology [59]. The traditional assessment of these patients often involves a fairly poorly tolerated "extended" defecographic technique, (colpocystodefecography), requiring opacification of the small bowel, bladder, vagina and even the peritoneal cavity to determine pathology of the pelvic floor compartments [60] with a presumptive interpretative process to define what radiologic finding represents the dominant pathology [61]. This approach has been supplemented where available by dynamic MRI imaging which appears to provide enhanced diagnosis of enteroceles [62] particularly in post-hysterectomy patients where there is variability in the routine use of culdosuspension [63].

Dynamic real-time TP-US represents a simpler more available alternative to dynamic MR imaging and is easily performed to assess the anterior, middle and posterior perineal and pelvic compartments providing clear high-resolution images of the anal canal, anal sphincters, puborectalis sling, bladder base, urethra and urethrovesical angle, vaginal vault and of the rectovaginal (rectogenital) septum. This novel technique has recently been reported by our group in an unselected group of patients presenting with a variety of anorectal disorders [12]. Our procedures are video-taped for orthograde and retrograde scrolling of dynamic images and static representative images may be used for clinical measurement. DTP-US is performed with a 7.5 MHz curvilinear transducer (B&K, Copenhagen) covered by a non-sterile latex glove with filling of the rectum and vagina with 50 mL of ultrasonographic coupling gel (Ultra-Gel: Aquarius 101; Medilab, USA) using a standard Luer syringe and a soft-end rubber catheter. For the complete procedure, 50 mL of Gastrografin (Schering, UK) diluted 1:1 with tap water may be ingested by the patient one hour prior to the procedure in order to visualize the small bowel.

The perineum of the patient is examined in the left-lateral position with systematic examination where the probe is placed firstly in a mid-sagittal plane on the perineal body to outline a general view of the pelvic floor and viscera and then rotated transversely onto the anus to define the posterior perineal structures in the axial dimension. Images of the infralevator viscera are obtained at rest, during maximal straining and with the patient asked to squeeze in order to prevent evacuation. Posterior perineal images show the anus and distal rectum and the anal sphincters are visualized using sagittal images of the anal canal and sphincter musculature which are identified by holding the transducer head in a plane in line with the vaginal introitus. Sagittal examination of the anterior perineum shows the distal vagina, bladder and urethra and is used to identify enteric loops, if present, between the rectal and vaginal walls in the territory of the rectovaginal septum, should the patient have an enterocele [64]. This technique has a substantial learning curve and requires considerable dedication, best in this author's view being performed by the surgeon with intimate knowledge of the anatomy and pathology of the region. The posture adopted by the patient during the examination is certainly not 'physiological' and the 'evacuation' of the gel can at best only reflect a simulated attempt at defecation which may fail to diagnose conditions where maximal straining at the end of defecation is clinically important, most notably, full-thickness rectal prolapse and rectoanal intussusception. The wide availability of these ultrasound probes, the lack of radiation, its ease of use, patient tolerance and low cost make this an attractive imaging modality in patients presenting with specialized and complex complaints to a pelvic floor unit.

Transvaginal ultrasonography has been relatively disappointing in the assessment of anorectal disease, being comparatively poor at demonstration of anterior fistula-in-ano, EAS defects and the definition of anatomical problems of the perineal body [65, 66]. The procedure may be performed with dedicated transvaginal (or endoanal) probes and may be combined with transintroital balloon sonography. The author's use of this modality has been limited to the delineation of certain low rectovaginal and anovaginal fistulae not detected on transperineal sonography as well as for assessment of masses presenting within the rectogenital septum [67].

In conclusion, the coloproctologist is the best practitioner to use and interpret ultrasonography in a referred proctologic practice and this represents an important clinical advance. Proctologic ultrasonography requires trainable skill in its basic performance and in the use of its ancillary modifications. These include contrast enhancement for the delineation of complex fistula tracks, 3-dimensional modifications for the stage assessment of rectal and anal tumors, dedicated ultrasound-guided biopsy probe use for confirmation of tumor recurrence after chemoradiation and of perirectal lymph nodes and transperineal techniques for the definition of complex fistulas, in the immediate postoperative period to image sphincteroplasties and perineoplasties, in the assessment of certain pediatric anorectal anomalies and for specialized use in complex symptomatic evacuatory disorders. The process of accreditation in the training of ultrasonography for the coloproctologist has not yet been formalized but this represents an area that Coloproctological Associations throughout the world will have to address in the context of specialized training programs.

References

1. Law PJ, Bartram CI (1989) Anal endosonography: technique and normal anatomy. Gastrointest Radiol 14:349-353
2. Beynon J, Foy DMA, Channer JL, Temple LN, Virjee J, Mortensen NJMCC (1986) The endosonic appearances of normal colon and rectum. Dis Colon Rectum 29:810-813
3. Burnett SJ, Bartram CI (1991) Endosonographic variations in the normal internal anal sphincter. Int J Colorect Dis 6:2-4
4. Papachrysostomou M, Pye SD, Wild SR, Smith AN (1993) Anal endosonography in asymptomatic subjects. Scand J Gastroenterol 28:551-556
5. Williams AB, Cheetham MJ, Bartram CI, Halligan S, Kamm MA, Nicholls RJ, Kmiot WA (2000) Gender differences in the longitudinal pressure profile of the anal canal related to anatomical structure as demonstrated on three-dimensional anal endosonography. Br J Surg 87:1674-1679
6. Dalley AF (1987) The riddle of the sphincters: the morphophysiology of the anorectal mechanisms reviewed. Am Surg 53:298-306
7. deSouza NM, Puni R, Zbar A, Gilderdale DJ, Koutts GA, Krausz T (1996) MR imaging of the anal sphincter in multiparous females using an endoanal coil: correlation with in vitro anatomy and appearances in fecal incontinence. Am J Roentgenol (AJR) 167:1465-1471
8. Zbar AP (2001) Magnetic resonance imaging and the coloproctologist. Tech Coloproctol 5:1-7
9. Lunniss PJ, Phillips RKS (1992) Anatomy and function of the anal longitudinal muscle. Br J Surg 79:882-884
10. Shafik AA (1976) A new concept of the anatomy of the anal sphincter mechanism and the physiology of defecation. IV. Anatomy of the perianal spaces. Invest Urol 13:424-428
11. Beer-Gabel M, Teshler M, Barzilai N, Lurie Y, Malnick S, Bass D, Zbar AP (2002) Dynamic

transperineal ultrasound in the diagnosis of pelvic floor disorders. Pilot study. Dis Colon Rectum 45:239-248
12. Beer-Gabel M, Teshler M, Schechtman E, Zbar AP (2004) Dynamic transperineal ultrasound versus defecography in patienst with evacuatory difficulty: a pilot study. Int J Colorect Dis 19:60-67
13. Wedemeyer J, Kirchhoff T, Sellge G, Bachmann O, Lotz J, Galanski M, Manns MP, Gebel MJ, Bleck JS (2004) Transcutaneous perianal sonography: a sensitive method for the detection of perianal inflammatory lesions in Crohn's disease. World J Gastroenterol 10:2859-2863
14. Mallouhi A, Bonatti H, Peer S, Lugger P, Conrad F, Bodner G (2004) Detection and characterization of perianal inflammatory disease. Accuracy of transperineal combined gray scale and color Doppler sonography. J Ultrasound Med 23:19-27
15. Goodsall DH (1900) Anorectal fistula. In: Diseases of the Anus and Rectum. Goodsall DH, Miles WE (eds) Longmans, Green & Co., London, pp 92-137
16. Martinez Hernandez Magro P, Villanueva Saenz E, Jaime Zavala M, Sandoval Munro RD, Rocha Ramirez JL (2003) Endoanal sonography in assessment of fecal incontinence following obstetric trauma. Ultrasound Obstet Gynecol 22:616-621
17. Garcia-Aguilar J, Pollack J, Lee SH, Hernandez de Anda E, Mellgren A, Wong WD, Finne CO, Rothenberger DA, Madoff RD (2002) Accuracy of endorectal ultrasonography in preoperative staging of rectal tumors. Dis Colon Rectum 45:10-15
18. Hunerbein M (2003) Endorectal ultrasound in rectal cancer. Colorectal Dis 5:402-405
19. Sangwan YP, Rosen L, Riether RD, Stasik JJ, Sheets JA, Khubchandani IT (1994) Is simple fistula-in-ano simple? Dis Colon Rectum 37:885-889
20. Schaffzin DM, Wong WD (2004) Surgeon performed ultrasound: endorectal ultrasound. Surg Clin N Am 84:1127-1149
21. Garcia-Aguilar J, Belmonte C, Wong WD, Goldberg SM, Madoff RD (1996) Anal fistula surgery: factors associated with recurrence and incontinence. Dis Colon Rectum 39:723-729
22. Parks AG, Gordon PH, Hardcastle JD (1976) A classification of fistula in ano. Br J Surg 63:1-12
23. Maccioni F, Colaiacomo MC, Stasolla A, Manganaro L, Izzo L, Marini M (2002) Value of MRI performed with phased-array coil in the diagnosis and pre-operative classification of perianal and anal fistulas. Radiol Med 104:58-67
24. Lunniss PJ, Kamm MA, Phillips RKS (1994) Factors affecting continence after surgery for anal fistula. Br J Surg 81:1382-1385
25. Cataldo PA, Senagore A, Luchtefeld MA (1993) Intrarectal ultrasound in the evaluation of perirectal abscesses. Dis Colon Rectum 36:554-558
26. Lengyel AJ, Hurst NG, Williams JG (2002) Pre-operative assessment of anal fistulas using endoanal ultrasound. Colorectal Dis 4:436-440
27. Barker PG, Lunniss PJ, Armstrong P, Reznek RH, Cottam K, Phillips RKS (1994) Magnetic resonance imaging of fistula-in-ano: technique, interpretation and accuracy. Clin Radiol 49:7-13
28. Spencer JA, Ward J, Ambrose NS (1998) Dynamic contrast-enhanced MR imaging of perianal fistulae. Clin Radiol 53:96-104
29. Maier AG, Funovics MA, Kreuzer SH, Herbst F, Wunderlich M, Teleky BK, Mittlbock M, Schima W, Lechner GL (2001) Evaluation of perianal sepsis:comparison of anal endosonography and magnetic resonance imaging. J Magn Reson Imaging 14:254-260
30. Stoker J, Hussain SM, van Kempen D, Elevelt AJ, Lameris JS (1996) Endoanal coil in MR imaging of anal fistulas. Am J Roetgenol (AJR) 166:360-362
31. West RL, Zimmerman DD, Dwarkasing S, Hussain SM, Hop WC, Schouten WR, Kuipers EJ, Felt-Bersma RJ (2003) Prospective comparison of hydrogen peroxide-enhanced three-dimensional endoanal ultrasonography and endoanal magnetic resonance imaging of perianal fistulas. Dis Colon Rectum 46:1407-1415
32. Chapple KS, Spencer JA, Windsor AC, Wilson D, Ward J, Ambrose NS (2000) Prognostic value of magnetic resonance imaging in the management of fistula-in-ano. Dis Colon Rectum 43:511-516
33. Ortiz H, Marzo J, Jimenez G, DeMiguel M (2002) Accuracy of hydrogen peroxide-enhanced ultrasound in the identification of internal openings of anal fistulas. Colorectal Dis 4:280-283

34. Moscowitz I, Baig MK, Nogueras JJ, Ovalioglu E, Weiss EG, Singh JJ, Wexner SD (2003) Accuracy of hydrogen peroxide enhanced endoanal ultrasonography in assessment of the internal opening of an anal fistula complex. Tech Coloproctol 7:133-137
35. Leroi AM, Kamm MA, Weber J, Denis P, Hawley PR (1997) Internal anal sphincter repair. Int J Colorectal Dis 12:243-245
36. Akbari H, Bernstein M (2005) Evaluation and management of postoperative faecal incontinence. In: Complex Anorectal Disorders; Investigation and Management. Wexner SD, Zbar AP, Pescatori M (eds). Springer Verlag, New York, pp 670-692
37. Yee LF, Birnbaum EH, Read TE, Kodner IJ, Fleshman JW (1999) Use of endoanal ultrasound in patients with rectovaginal fistula. Dis Colon Rectum 42:1057-1064
38. Pinedo G, Phillips RKS (1998) Labial fat pad grafts (modified Martius graft) in complex perianal fistulas. Ann R Coll Surg Engl 80:410-412
39. Solomon MJ, McLeod RS, Cohen EK, Cohen Z (1995) Anal wall thickness in normal and inflammatory conditions of the anorectum. Am J Gastroenterol 90:574-578
40. Dagli U, Over A, Tezel A, Ulker A, Temucin G (1999) Transrectal ultrasound in the diagnosis and management of inflammatory bowel disease. Endoscopy 31:152-157
41. Buchanan GN, Bartram CI, Williams AB, Halligan S, Cohen CR (2005) Value of hydrogen peroxide enhancement of three-dimensional endoanal ultrasound in fistula-in-ano. Dis Colon Rectum 48:141-147
42. Bonatti H, Lugger P, Hechenleitner P, Oberwalder M, Kafka-Ritsch R, Conrad F, Aigner F, Mallouhi A, Bodner G (2003) Transperineal sonography in anorectal disorders. Ultraschalle in Med 24:111-115
43. Sultan AH, Kamm MA, Hudson CN, Thomas JM, Bartram CI (1993) Anal-sphincter disruption during vaginal delivery. N Engl J Med 329:1905-1911
44. Damon H, Henry L, Barth X, Mion F (2002) Fecal incontinence in females with a past history of vaginal delivery: significance of anal sphincter defects detected by ultrasound. Dis Colon Rectum 45:1445-1450
45. Allen RF, Hosker GL, Smith AR, Wardell DW (1990) Pelvic floor damage and childbirth: a neurophysiological study. Br J Obstet Gynaecol 97:770-779
46. Sultan AH, Nicholls RJ, Kamm MA (1993) Anal endosonography and correlation with in vitro and in vivo anatomy. Br J Surg 80:508-511
47. Bollard RC, Gardiner A, Lindow S, Phillips RKS, Duthie GS (2002) Normal female anal sphincter: difficulties in interpretation explained. Dis Colon Rectum 45:171-175
48. de Parades V, Etienney I, Thabut D, Beaulieu S, Tank M, Assemekang B, Marié V, Toubia MK, Wehbe A, Mosnier H, Gadonneix P, Harvey T, Atienza P (2004) Anal sphincter injury after forceps delivery: myth or reality. A prospective ultrasound study of 93 females. Dis Colon Rectum 47:24-34
49. Briel JV, Stoker J, Rociu E, Lameris JS, Hop WC, Schouten WR (1999) External anal sphincter atrophy on endoanal MR imaging adversely affects outcome after sphincteroplasty. Br J Surg 86:3122-3127
50. Giordano P, Remzi A, Efron J, Gervaz P, Weiss EG, Nogueras JJ, Wexner SD (2002) Previous sphincter repair does not affect the outcome of repeat repair. Dis Colon Rectum 45:635-640
51. Gold DM, Bartram CI, Halligan S, Humphries KN, Kamm MA, Kmiot WA (1999) 3-dimensional endoanal sonography in assessing anal canal injury. Br J Surg 86:365-370
52. Zbar AP, Beer-Gabel M, Chiappa AC, Aslam M (2001) Fecal incontinence after minor anorectal surgery. Dis Colon Rectum 44:1610-1623
53. Zbar AP, Aslam M, Allgar V (2000) Faecal incontinence after internal sphincterotomy for anal fissure. Tech Coloproctol 4:25-28
54. Abbasakoor F, Nelson M, Beynon J, Patel B, Carr ND (1998) Anal endosonography in patients with anorectal symptoms after haemorrhoidectomy. Br J Surg 85:1522-1524
55. Zimmerman DD, Gosselink MP, Hop WC, Darby M, Briel JW, Schouten WR (2003) Impact of two different types of anal retractor on fecal continence after fistula repair: a prospective, randomized, clinical trial. Dis Colon Rectum 46:1674-1679
56. Ho YH, Tsang C, Tang CL, Nyam D, Eu KW, Seow-Choen F (2000) Anal sphincter injuries from stapling instruments introduced transanally. Dis Colon Rectum 43:169-173

57. Ho YH, Seow-Choen F, Tsang C, Eu KW (2001) Randomized trial assessing anal sphincter injuries after stapled haemorrhoidectomy. Br J Surg 88:1449-1455
58. Maglinte DD, Kelvin FM, Fitzgerald K, Hale DS, Benson T (1999) Association of compartment defects in pelvic floor dysfunction. Am J Roentgenol (AJR) 172:439-444
59. Kenton K, Shott S, Brubaker L (1999) The anatomic and functional variability of rectocele in women. Int Urogynecol J Pelvic Floor Dysfunct 10:96-99
60. Kelvin FM, Hale DS, Maglinte DD, Patten BJ, Benson JT (1999) Female pelvic organ prolapse: diagnostic contribution of dynamic cystoproctography and comparison with physical examination. Am J Roentgenol (AJR) 173:31-37
61. Siproudhis L, Robert A, Vilotte J, Bretagne JF, Heresbach D, Raoul JL, Gosselin M (1993) How accurate is clinical examination in diagnosing and quantifying pelvirectal disorders? A prospective study in a group of 50 patients complaining of defecatory difficulties. Dis Colon Rectum 36:430-438
62. Lienemann A, Anthuber C, Baron A, Reiser M (2000) Diagnosing enteroceles using dynamic magnetic resonance imaging. Dis Colon Rectum 43:205-213
63. Comiter CV (2001) Repair of enterocele and vault prolapse: transvaginal culdosuspension Tech Urol 7:146-151
64. Beer-Gabel M, Frudinger A, Zbar AP (2005) Ultrasound in coloproctologic practice: dynamic transperineal ultrasound and transvaginal sonography. In: Complex Anorectal Disorders: Investigation and Management. Wexner SD, Zbar AP, Pescatori M (eds) Springer Verlag, London, pp 246-262
65. Sultan AH, Loder PB, Bartram CI, Kamm MA, Hudson CN (1994) Vaginal endosonography: new approach to image the undisturbed anal sphincter. Dis Colon Rectum 37:1296-1299
66. Stewart L, Wilson SR (1999) Transvaginal sonography of the anal sphincter: reliable or not? Am J Roentgenol (AJR) 173:179-185
67. Aigner F, Zbar AP, Ludwikowski B, Kreczy A, Kovacs P, Fritsch H (2004) The rectogenital septum: morphology, function, and clinical relevance. Dis Colon Rectum 47:131-140

2 Clinical Use of Two-Dimensional Endoanal and Transvaginal Sonography

Mario Pescatori • Stella Ayabaca • Maria Spyrou • Paola De Nardi

Introduction

Endoanal ultrasonography has an established place in benign proctological practice, specifically in the assessment of external and internal anal sphincter defects in patients presenting with fecal incontinence, in perirectal sepsis, (either of cryptogenic or other origin) and in some patients presenting with evacuatory difficulty where extrarectal lesions resulting in mechanical block are demonstrated [1-5]. It may also prove useful in specialized conditions referred to a proctology clinic, including paradoxical puborectalis contraction (anismus), solitary rectal ulcer syndrome and rectal prolapse, as well as in difficult cases of persistent proctalgia. Specific examples of its use in a tertiary referral practice are shown below with all patients being assessed (unless otherwise stated) in the Sims left lateral position* utilizing a 7.5 MHz endoanal probe (B-K, Copenhagen DK).

The role of transvaginal sonography in proctological practice appears to be limited. Hopes that it would adequately demonstrate the soft-tissue structures of the perineal body have proven fruitless and it is now recommended in situations where there is endoanal luminal distortion preventing utilization of an endoanal probe [6, 7]. In some specialist circumstances there is a complementary advantage in transvaginal ultrasound for some anteriorly disposed fistulae-in-ano as well as for the definition of anovaginal fistulae [8]. The delineation of anterior defects in the external anal sphincter and for the postoperative follow-up of anterior sphincteroplasty has proven relatively poor [9-11].

* In this chapter, ultrasound image display has the same orientation so that the left side of the patient corresponds to the lower edge of the monitor while his back is seen on the left side of the screen. MRI images are with the patients in supine position. Operative field images are with the patients in lithotomy position.

Normal Anatomy (Endoanal and Transvaginal)

Figure 1 shows the normal anatomy obtained using this probe, with the traditionally hyperechoic internal anal sphincter (IAS), the hyperechoic external anal sphincter (EAS) and the typically hyperechoic longitudinal muscle (a continuation of the longitudinal muscle layer of the rectum) as seen variably in patients. The natural tendency is for the IAS to generally enlarge its axial dimensions with age and for the rostral extent of the sphincter musculature to be greater in males in comparison with females [12].

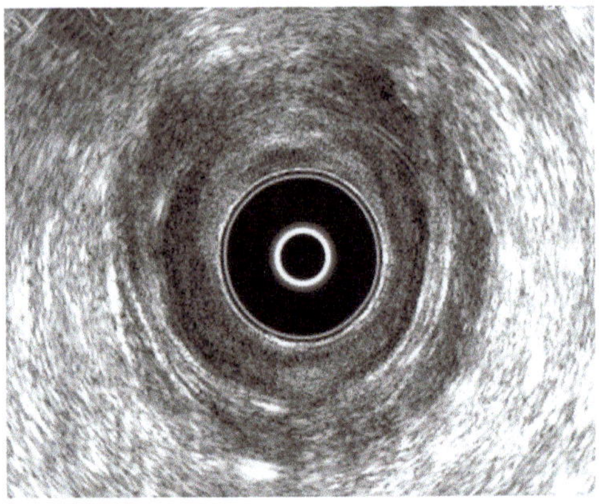

Fig. 1a. Endoanal ultrasound (high anal canal). The distinctive presence of the U-shaped puborectalis sling is the main landmark

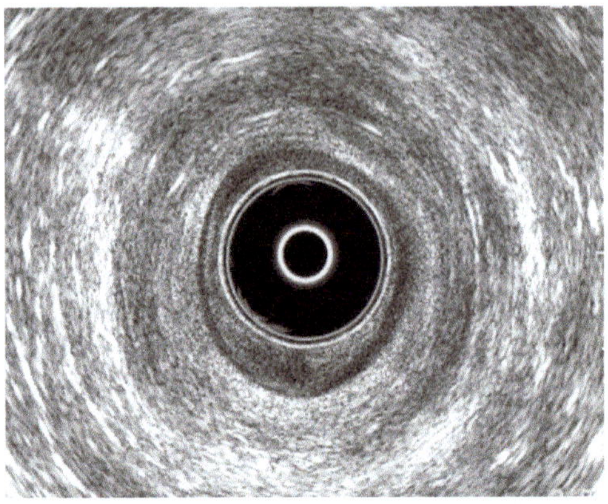

Fig. 1b. Lower anal canal. The lower end of the hypoechoic internal anal sphincter virtually disappears to leave only the terminal subcutaneous portion of the hyperechoic external anal sphincter appearing as a defined bright ring

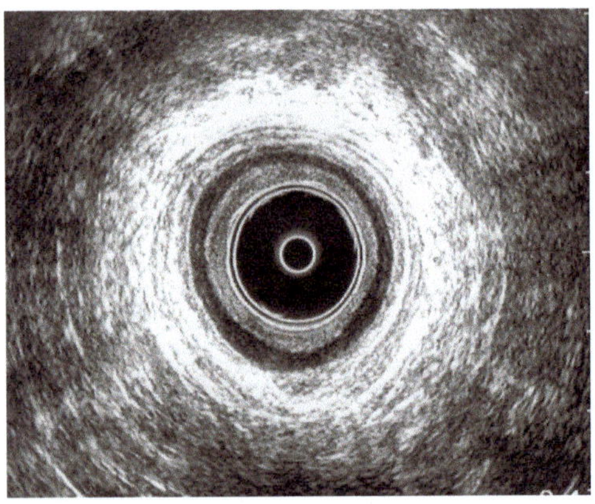

Fig. 1c. Endoanal ultrasound of the mid anal canal showing the hypoechoic internal anal sphincter and the hyperechoic external anal sphincter. In some patients there is evidence of a well formed longitudinal muscle which is a continuation of the longitudinal muscle coat of the rectum

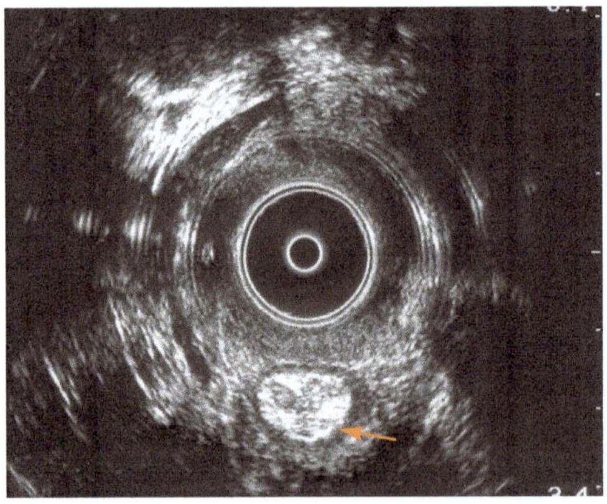

Fig. 1d. Transvaginal ultrasound. The external and internal sphincter complexes are imaged; within the internal sphincter lies the internal haemorrhoidal plexus (*arrow*). Patients are in lithotomy position

Anal Sepsis

Anal Abscess

The vast majority of simple perirectal sepsis (abscesses and fistulae) do not require specialized imaging [13]. In those patients with unexpected recurrent sepsis, non-cryptogenic sepsis, associated immunosuppression or where there is an associated history of irradition, it is wise to assess the perirectal sepsis by specialized imaging. Here, ultrasonography may be limited when there is translevator extension of an abscess, as the endoanal probe is unable to adequately couple above the puborectalis. This is of importance also when it may be deemed that a collection of pus presenting in the ischiorectal space is actually generated from above the pelvic floor. In this circumstance, injudicious drainage of the abscess through the ischiorectal fossa will inevitably result in a high extrasphincteric fistula [14]. Moreover, certain tracks and collections which lie beyond the focal distance of the endorectal probe (including some rectovaginal fistulae) will be difficult to detect with any endorectal ultrasonic assembly. In these two circumstances, if high quality soft-tissue resolution magnetic resonance imaging (MRI) is available, this will prove essential in defining the anatomy of complex fistulous disease in order to successfully eradicate the problem. This approach may be coupled with endorectal sonography to assess the presence of the secondary effects of destructive perirectal sepsis which may require reconstructive surgery in their own right; namely, an assessment of the internal and external anal sphincters, definition of the integrity of the perineal body and exclusion of an ano- or rectovaginal fistula.

Transvaginal probes are uncommonly used as adjuncts in perirectal sepsis. They may have limited value in some anterior abscesses as well as, defining low anovaginal fistulae, particularly in patients with perianal Crohn's disease where there is anal distortion or discomfort preventing adequate placement of the endoanal probe assembly. It can also prove of value in some patients with a deficient perineal body in its delineation of the rectovaginal septum where perineoplasty is contemplated and where transperineal sonography may prove more difficult to interpret.

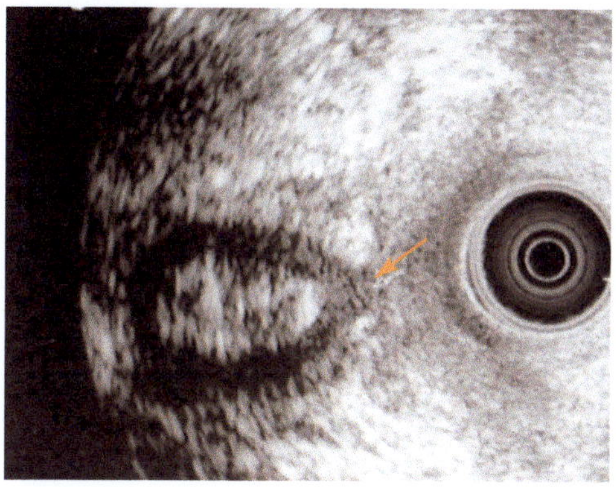

Fig. 2. Transvaginal ultrasound showing a low anterior intersphincteric abscess (*arrow*)

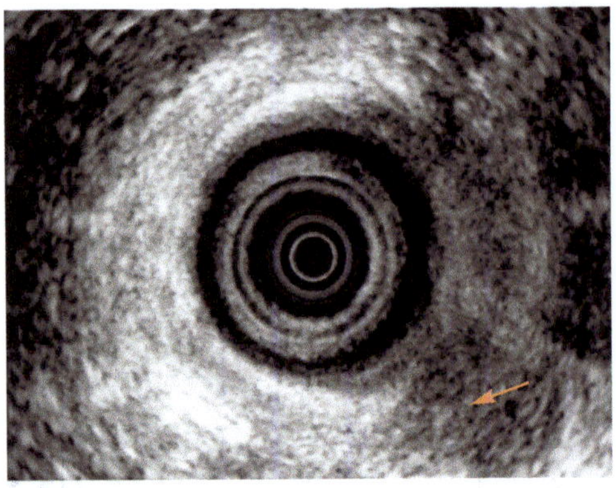

Fig. 3a. High left-sided intersphincteric collection (*arrow*)

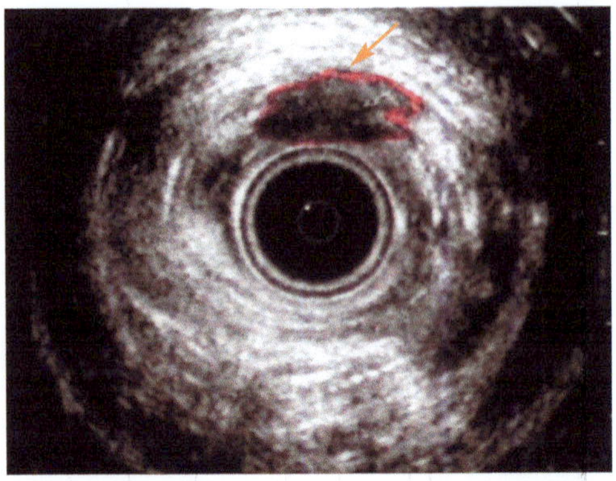

Fig. 3b. Right anal horseshoe extension in the subcutaneous plane in the same case (*arrow*)

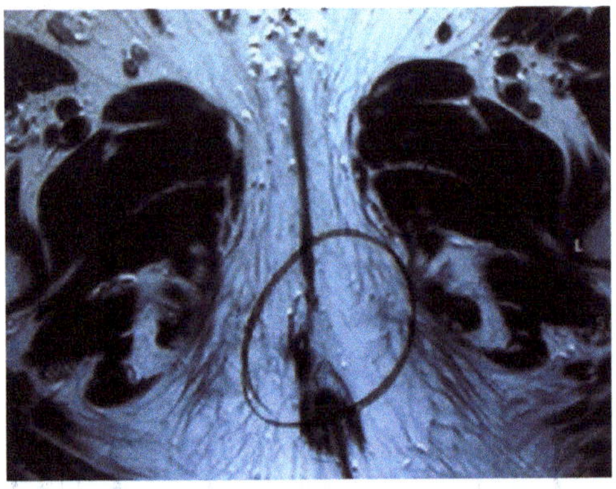

Fig. 3c. T2-weighted magnetic resonance image (coronal view) of the same case showing an infralevator collection (*circled*)

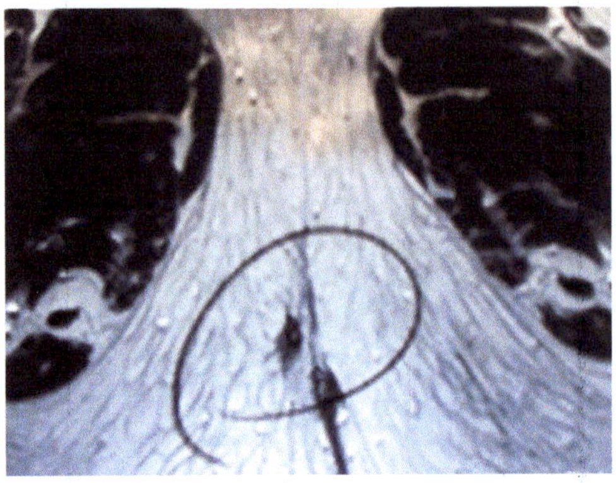

Fig. 3d. T2-weighted MRI: perianal fistula. Ultrasound: Sims position. MRI: supine position

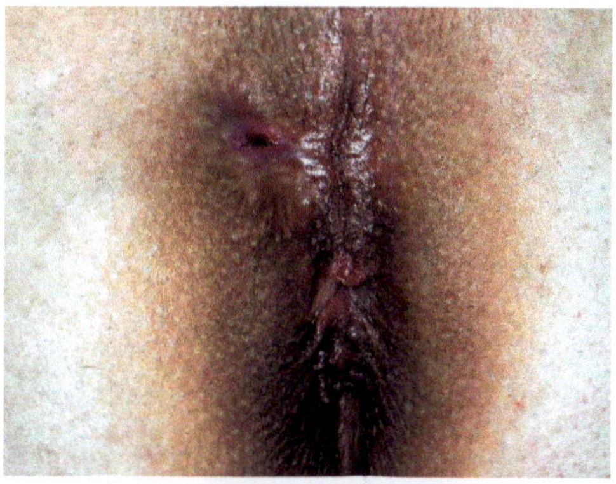

Fig. 3e. Operative field of the same case: external opening in the right antero-lateral perianal skin

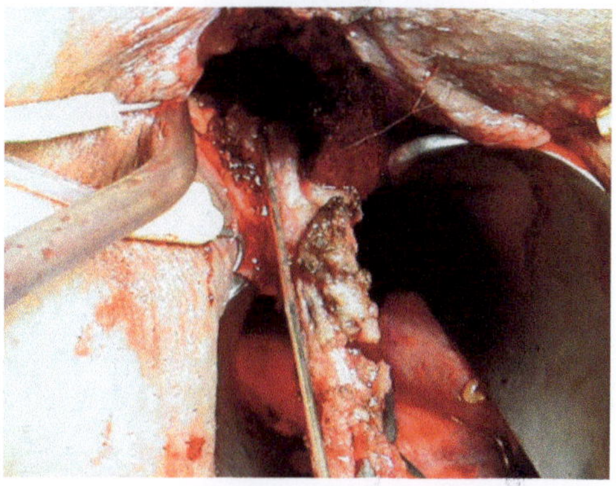

Fig. 3f. Excision of the underlying inter-sphincteric fistula

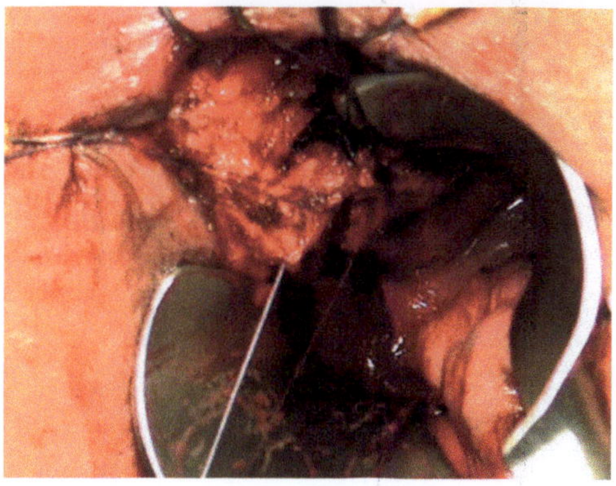

Fig. 3g. Drainage of the associated abscess

Intersphincteric Abscess

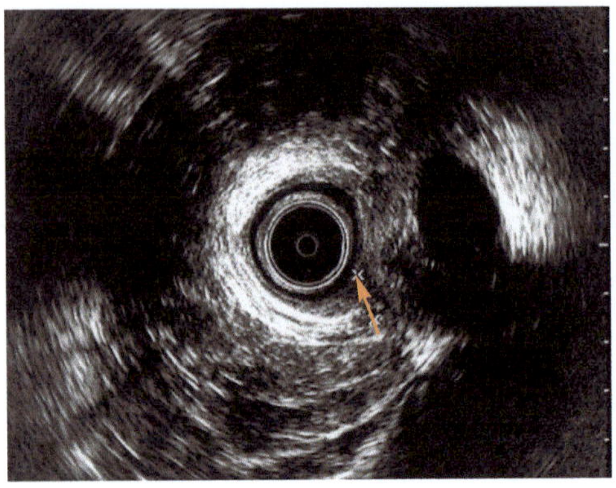

Fig. 4a. Anterolateral intersphincteric abscess (*arrow*) evident in the upper anal canal at the level of the hyperechoic puborectalis sling

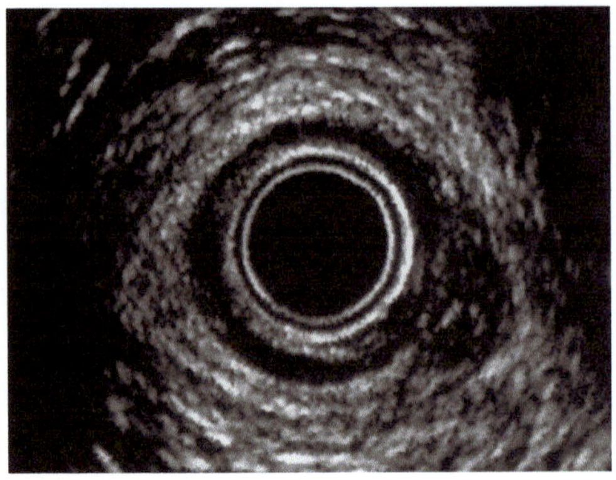

Fig. 4b. Intersphincteric abscess in the middle anal canal

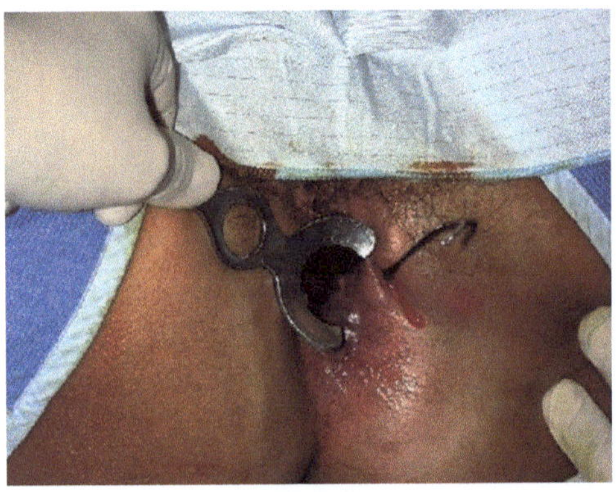

Fig. 4c. At operation, the intersphincteric fistula is probed

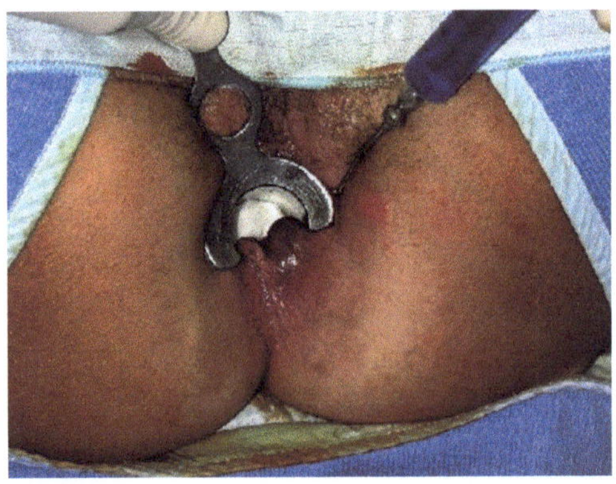

Fig. 4d. Methylene blue injection is used to look for communication with the anal canal

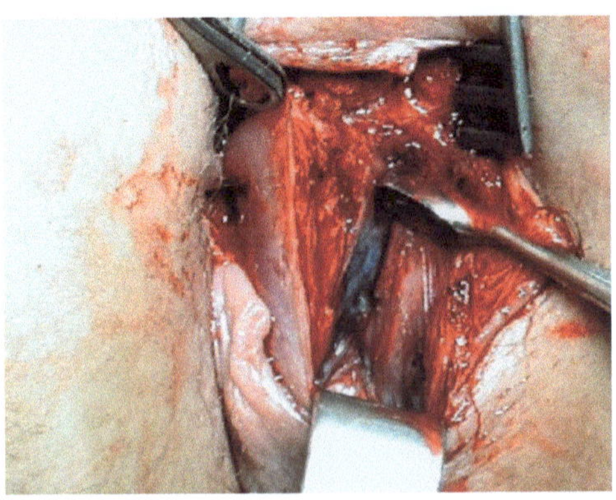

Fig. 4e. Curettage of the abscess

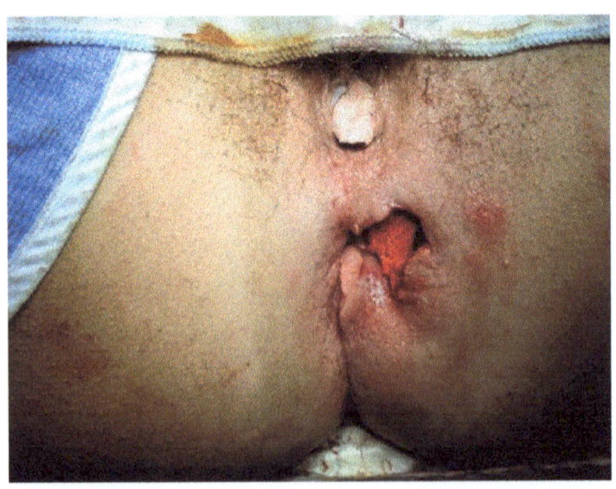

Fig. 4f. Marsupialized final perianal surgical wound

Chronic Perirectal Sepsis

Deep-seated recurrent or residual cryptogenic sepsis may be clinically difficult to detect where there is substantial endoanal scarring with poor appreciation of horseshoe abscess formation. Here endoanal sonography will assist in the definition of intersphincteric abscess collections which may encircle the anal canal either in the infralevator or supralevator plane. In some cases, surface MR imaging is required to define those situations where the origin of the sepsis is pelvirectal, breaking through the levator plate and presenting in the ischiorectal fossa. In this circumstance, drainage will inevitably result in an extrasphincteric fistula and distinction must be made from those patients presenting with a primary ischiorectal abscess with supralevator extension where the correct treatment is ischiorectal drainage [14].

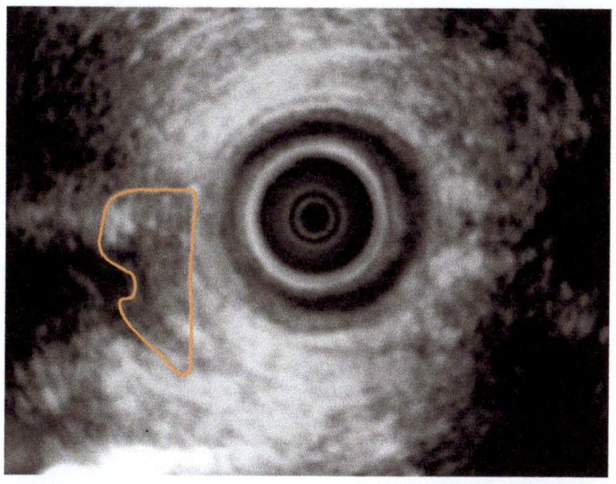

Fig. 5a. Preoperative anal ultrasound showing a chronic posterior and left lateral abscess pocket (*marked*)

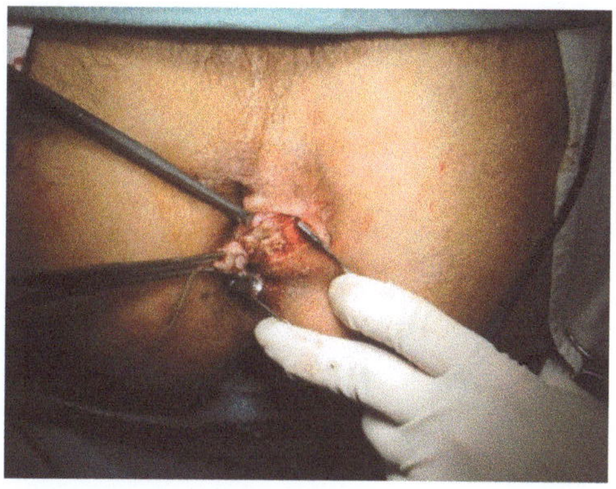

Fig. 5b. Operative field of the same patient with an intersphincteric approach

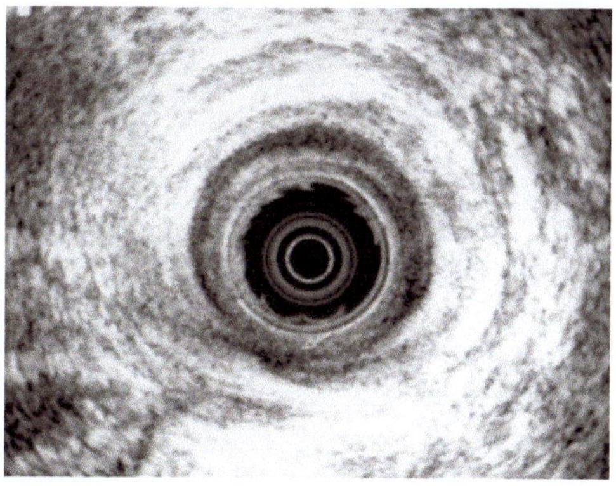

Fig. 5c. Postoperative fibrosis (a posterior area of mixed echogenicity) in the same patient

Perianal Abscess Following Hemorrhoidectomy

Deep seated (or superficial) perirectal sepsis may on occasion be responsible for poor functional outcomes and persistent anal pain following a conventional hemorrhoidectomy [15].

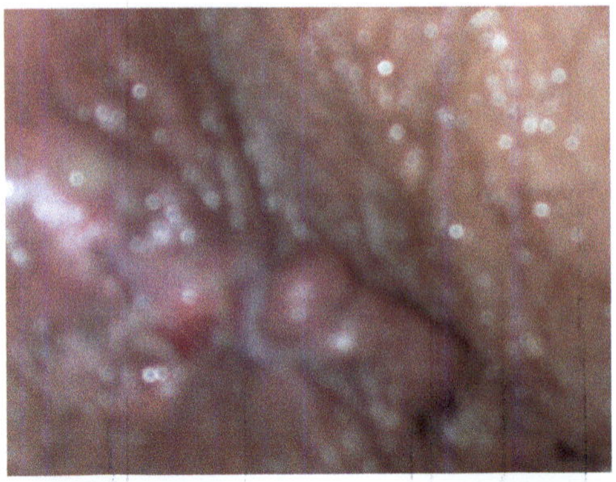

Fig. 6a. An external orifice with pus is evident after an open hemorrhoidectomy wound. In this case an endoanal ultrasound probe was unable to be used because of patient pain

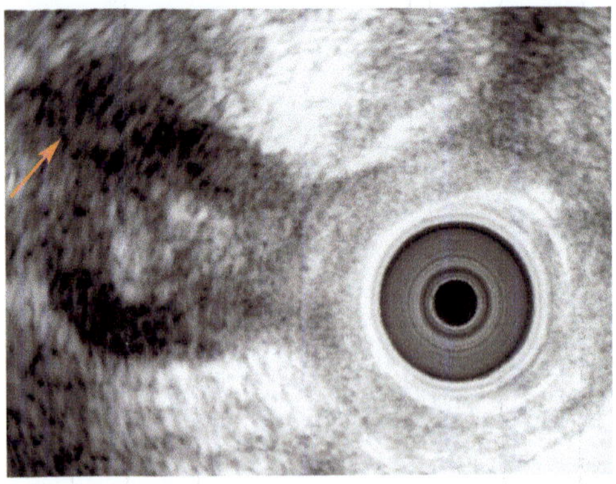

Fig. 6b. Transvaginal sonography was able to demonstrate a low intersphincteric abscess (*arrow*)

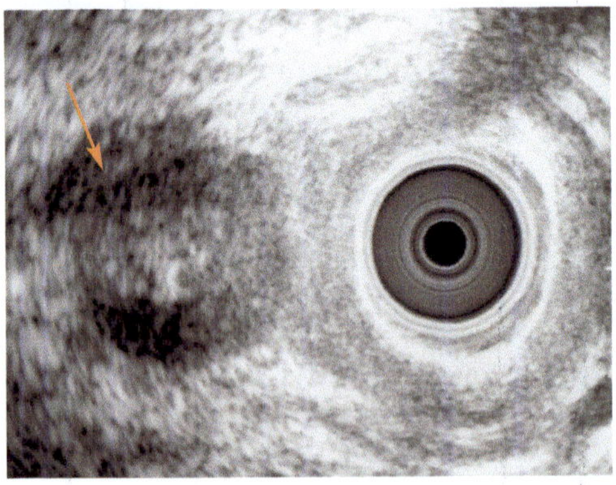

Fig. 6c. Transvaginal ultrasound showing intersphincteric abscess in a more superficial plane (*arrow*)

Intersphincteric Fistula

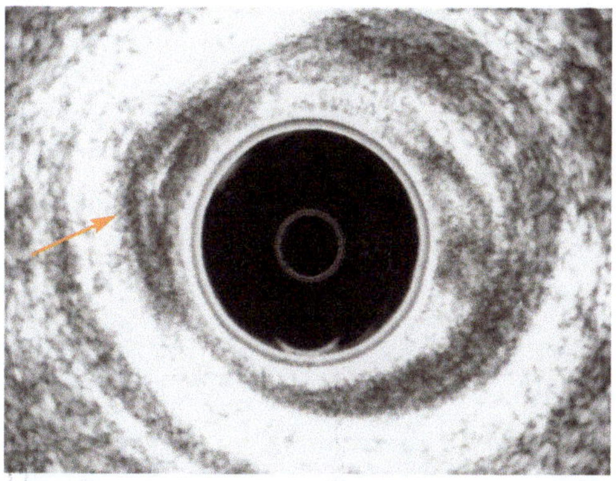

Fig. 7a. An endoanal ultrasound showing a low intersphincteric posterior fistula (*arrow*)

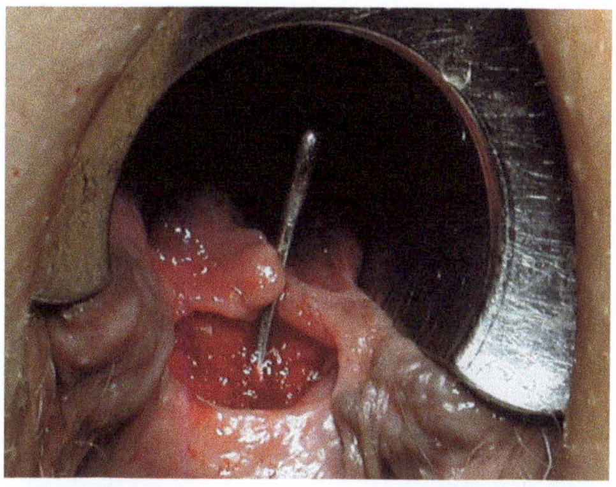

Fig. 7b. Intraoperative probing of the fistula in this case

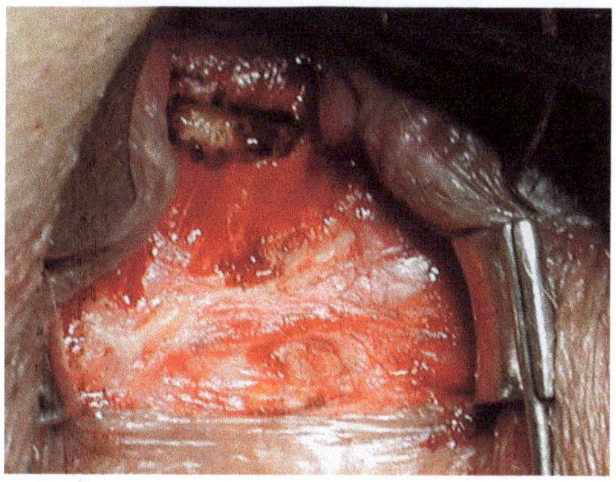

Fig. 7c. Formal fistulotomy

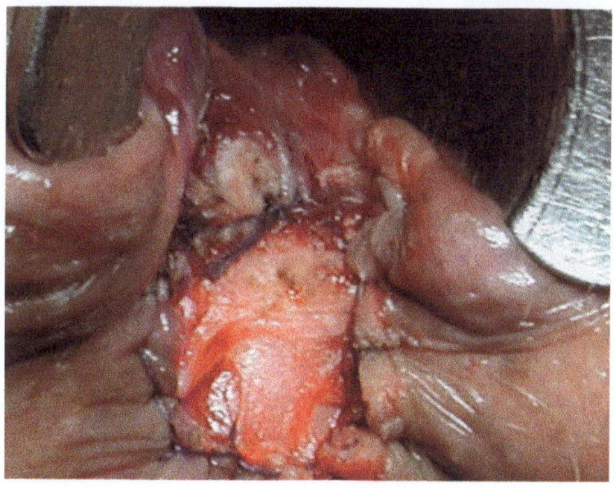

Fig. 7d. Marsupialization of the wound

Trans-Sphincteric Fistula

Preoperative (or intraoperative sonography) either alone or hydrogen peroxide-enhanced will define the presence of an underlying fistula in patients presenting with primary abscess collections as well as the adherence to Goodsall's rule, associated secondary tracks and collections, significant horseshoeing (either in the retrorectal or anteroanal planes) and the relationship of the collections and/or tracks to the main levator plane. Secondary information of great importance to the coloproctologist include the presence of destructive damage to the internal and/or external anal sphincters, perineal body destruction and the presence of an associated ano- or rectovaginal fistula. Each of these secondary features of destructive perirectal sepsis may require reconstrucitve surgery in their own right.

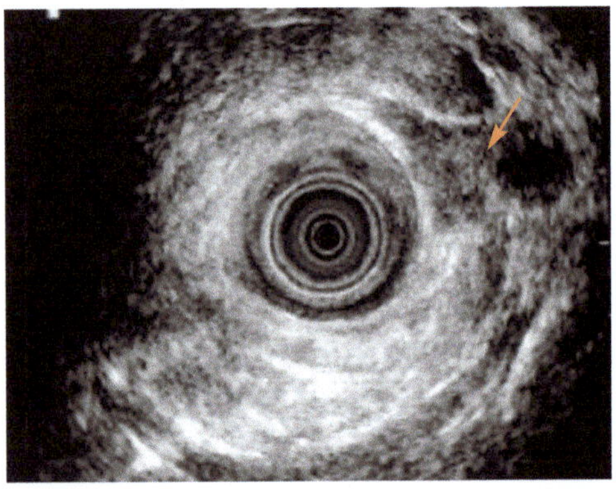

Fig. 8a. Anterior fistula and concomitant abscess (*arrow*)

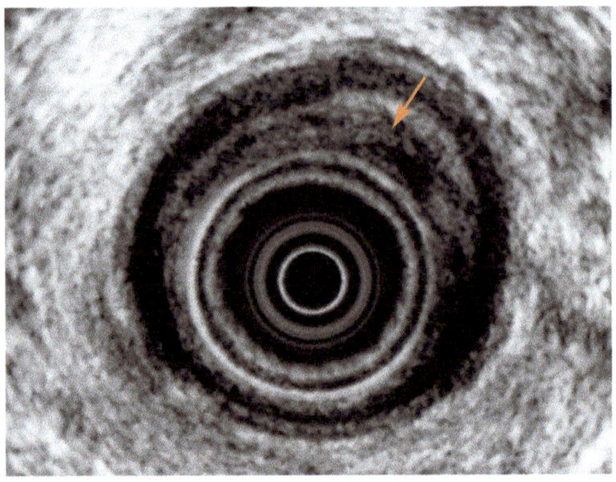

Fig. 8b. Simultaneous hemorrhoids in the same patient (*arrow*)

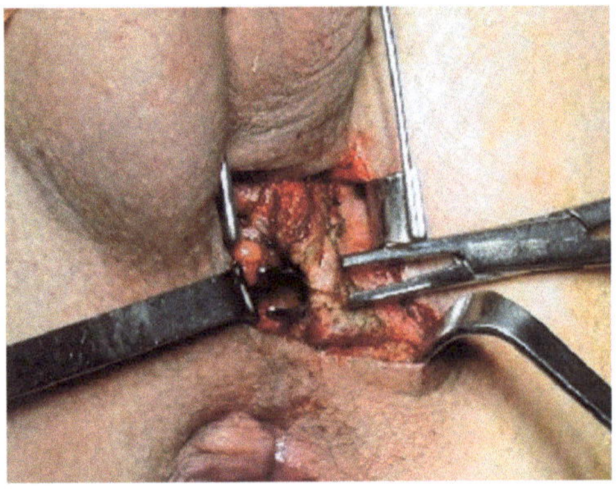

Fig. 8c. Operative field of the same patient showing the intersphincteric dissection of the fistula

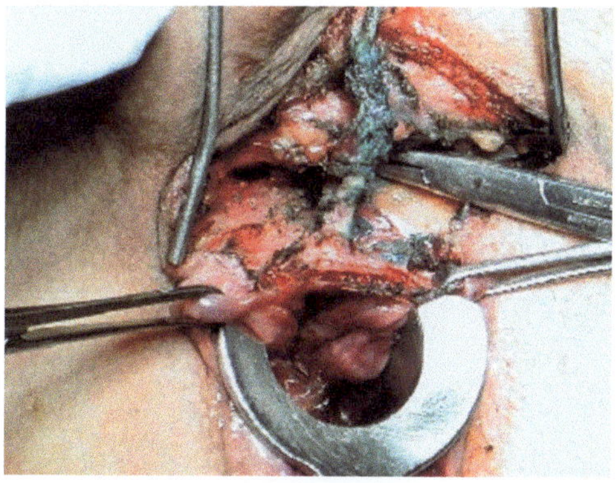

Fig. 8d. Operative steps of the fistulectomy. Internal opening of the fistula

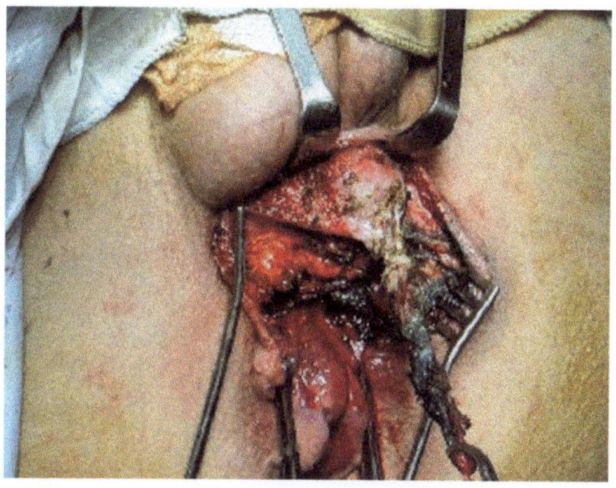

Fig. 8e. The fistulous track has been cored out

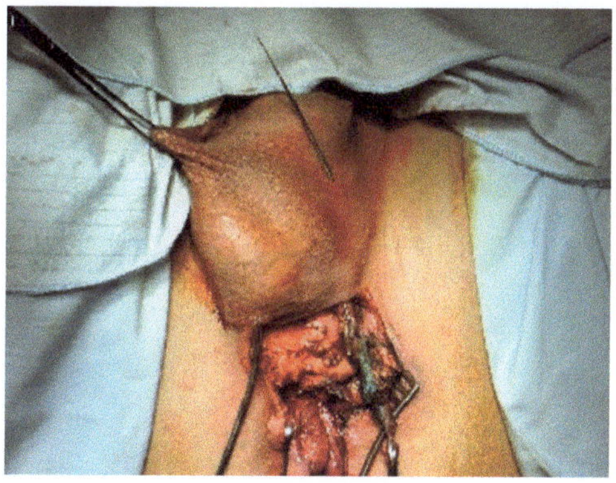

Fig. 8f. Wound at the end of fistulectomy

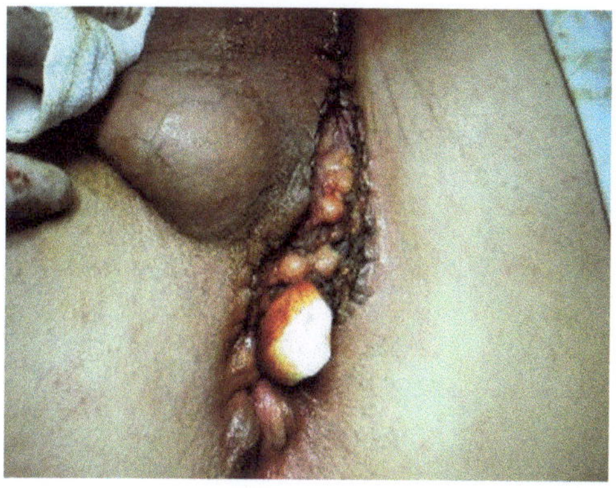

Fig. 8g. Terminal marsupialization of the resultant wound

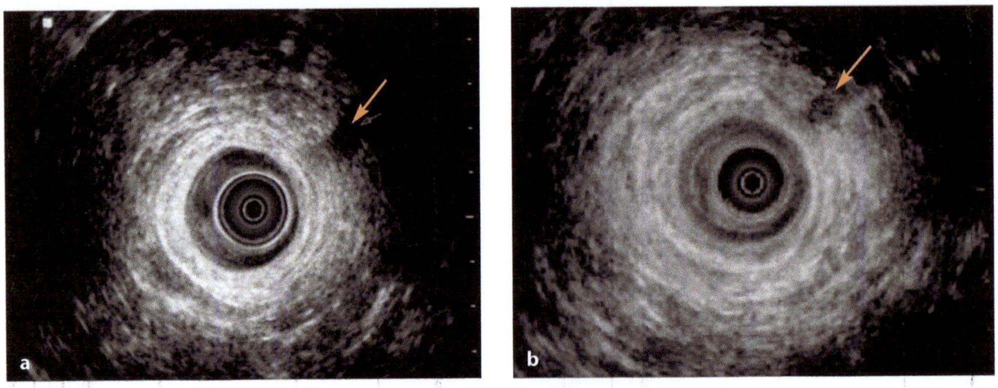

Fig. 9a, b. Trans-sphincteric fistula (*arrows*). Preoperative endoanal ultrasound

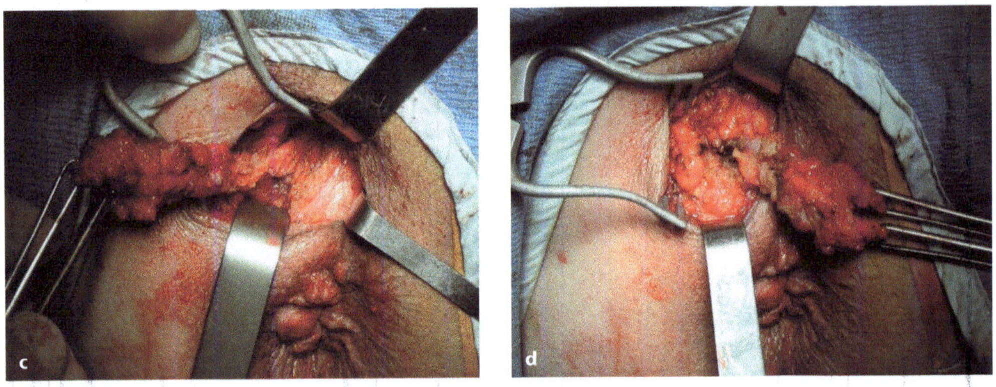

Fig. 9c, d. Operative fistulectomy of the same case: the fistulous track has been excised and held by forceps

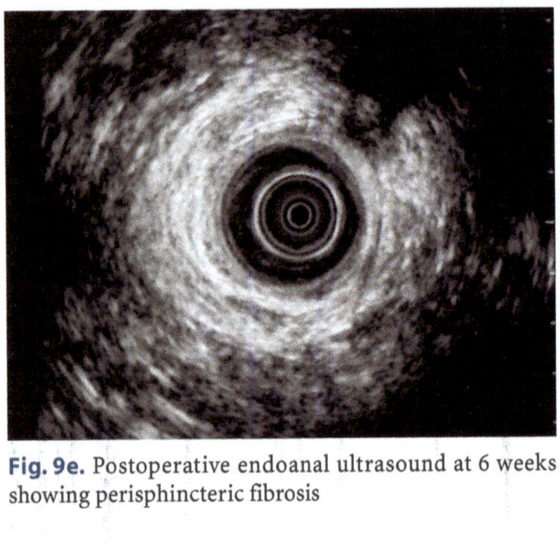

Fig. 9e. Postoperative endoanal ultrasound at 6 weeks showing perisphincteric fibrosis

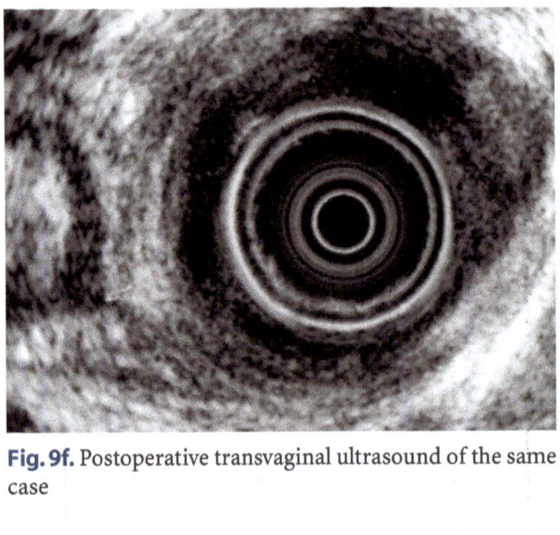

Fig. 9f. Postoperative transvaginal ultrasound of the same case

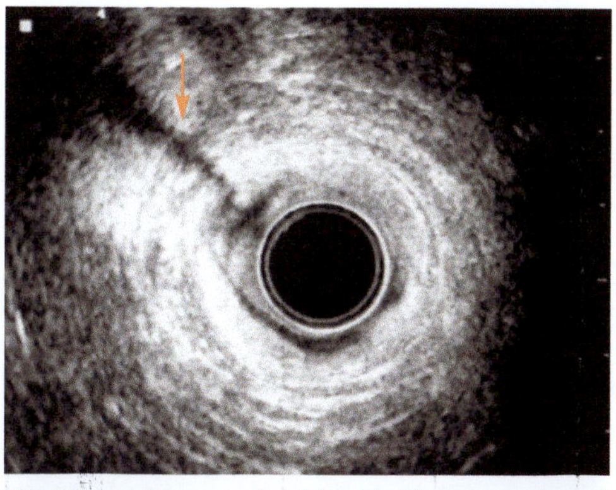

Fig. 10. Another case of a right-sided low posterolateral trans-sphincteric fistula (*arrow*)

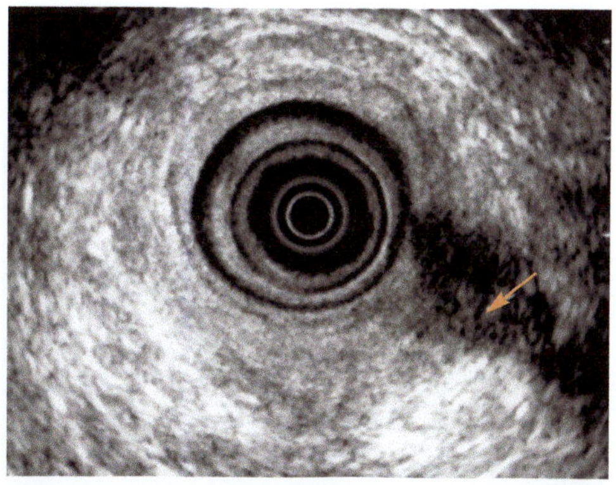

Fig. 11. An anterolateral left-sided trans-sphincteric fistula with concomitant abscess (*arrow*)

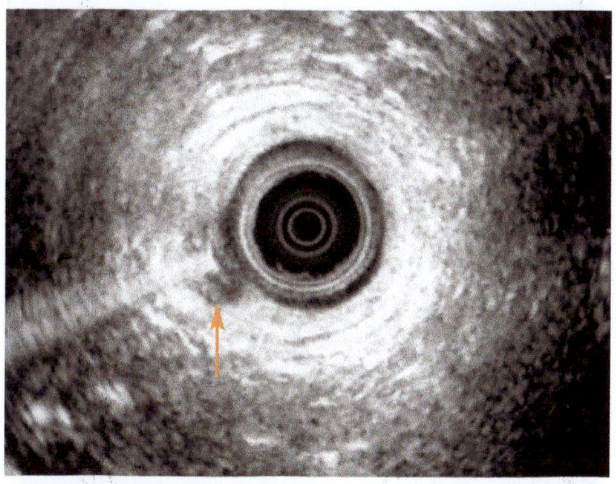

Fig. 12. Intraoperative endoanal ultrasound of a posterior low trans-sphincteric fistula confirmed by an indwelling Lockhart-Mummery probe, with a corresponding intersphincteric abscess (*arrow*)

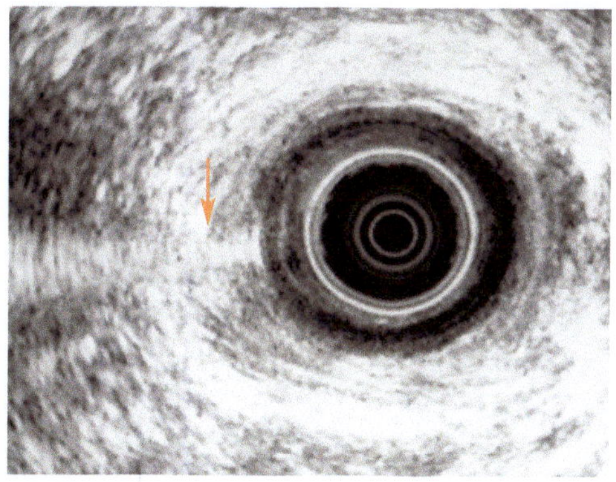

Fig. 13. A low posterior trans-sphincteric fistula crossing the superficial portion of the external anal sphincter (*arrow*)

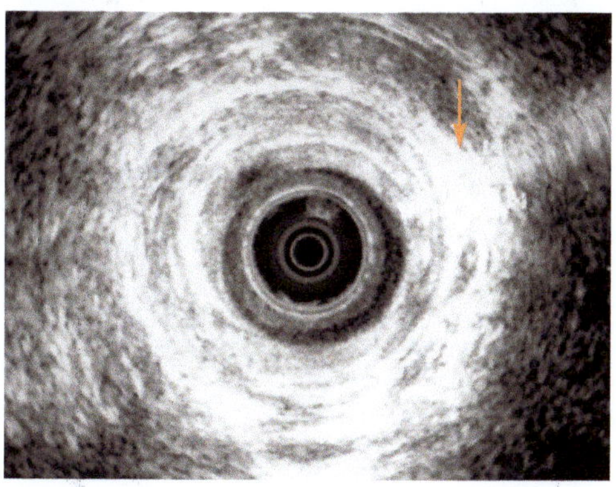

Fig. 14. A low anterior trans-sphincteric fistula crossing the superficialis portion of the external anal sphincter (*arrow*)

Recurrent Trans-Sphincteric Fistula

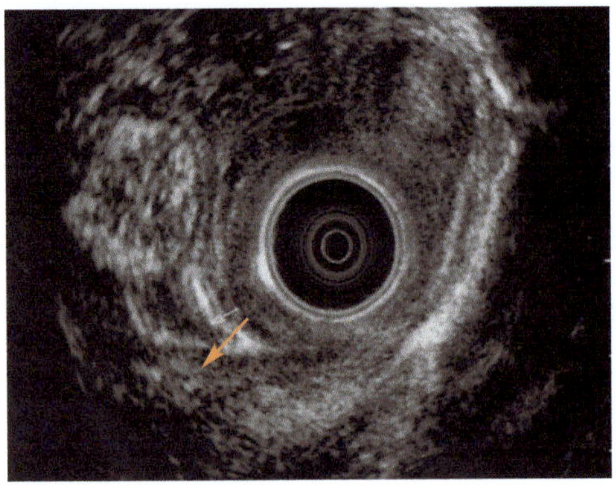

Fig. 15a. Transvaginal ultrasound in a 47 year-old patient with a recurrent ischiorectal abscess (*arrow*)

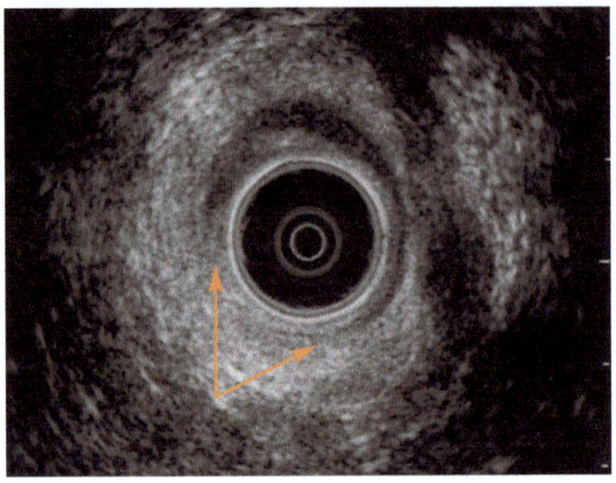

Fig. 15b. Endoanal ultrasonography of the lower anal canal in the same patient with evidence of a post-surgical defect of the internal anal sphincter (*arrows*) between the 2 and 6 o'clock positions

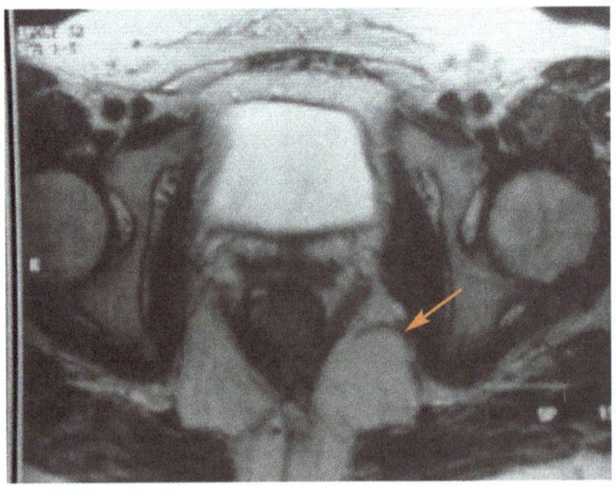

Fig. 15c. Axial MRI of the same patient showing the trans-sphincteric fistula (*arrow*)

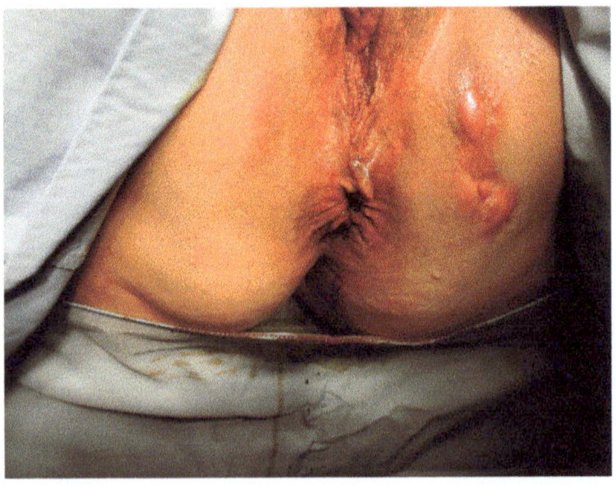

Fig. 15d. Clinical appearance of the principal perianal abscess and external opening of the fistula

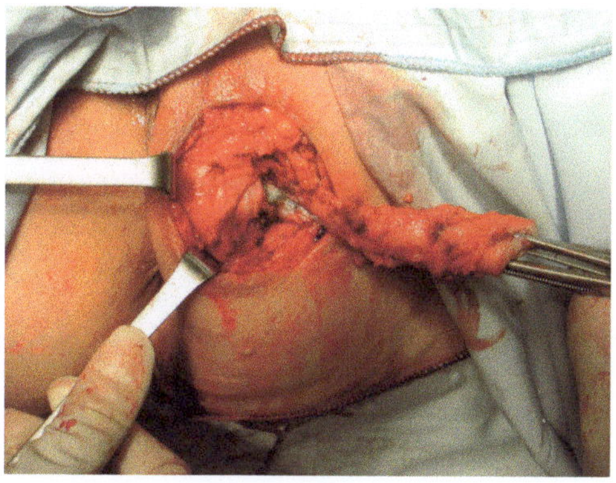

Fig. 15e. Operative fistulectomy

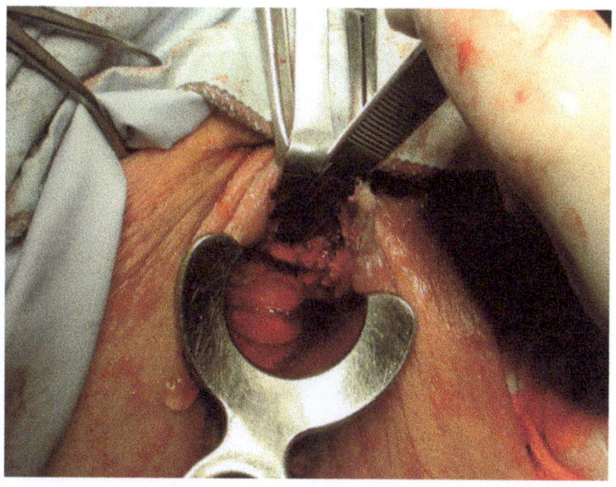

Fig. 15f. In this case an internal sphincterotomy was initially performed to drain the intersphincteric plane

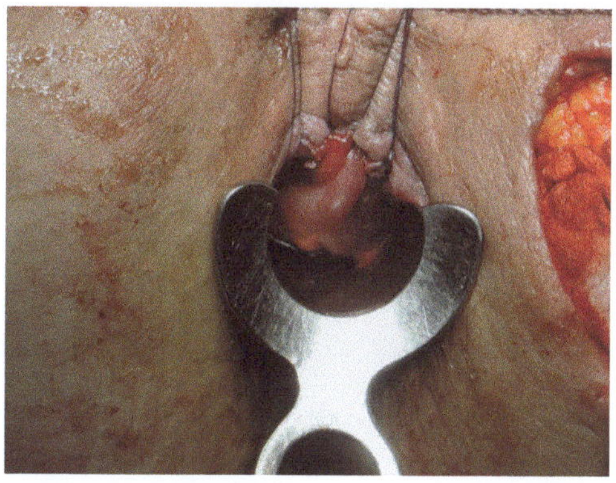

Fig. 15g. A rectal advancement flap was created as definitive treatment after sphincter repair

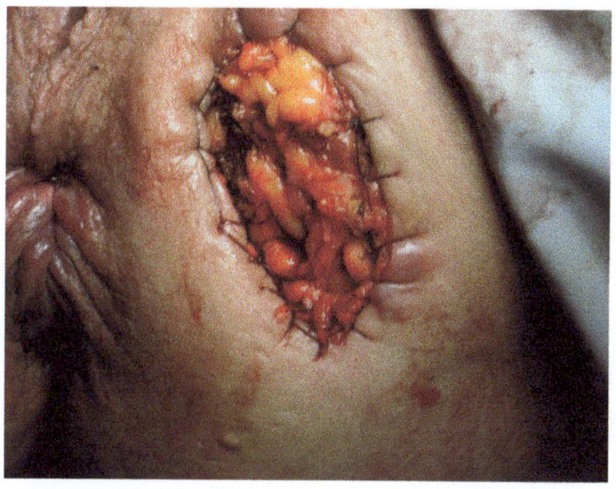

Fig. 15h. Marsupialization of the abscess wound was employed in this case

High Trans-Sphincteric Fistula with Ischiorectal and Deep Retroanal Abscess

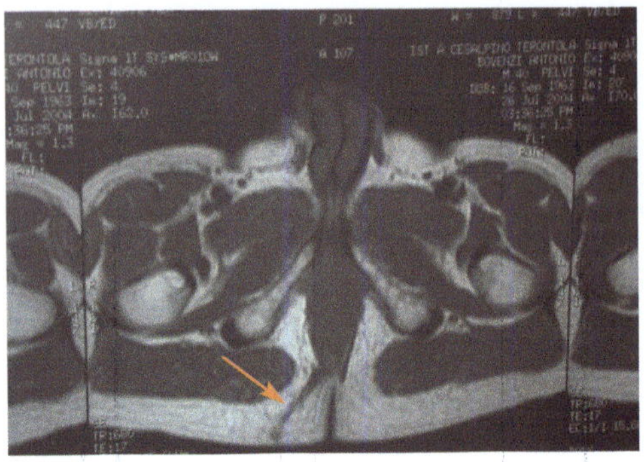

Fig. 16a. Axial T2-weighted MRI showing a high trans-sphincteric fistula (*arrow*). There was no evidence of a primary pelvirectal origin

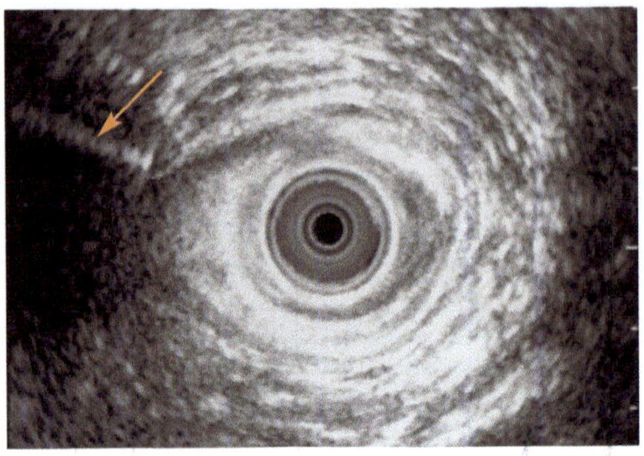

Fig. 16b. Endoanal ultrasound of the same patient confirming the trans-sphincteric fistula. A probe has been inserted into the superficial part of the track (*arrow*)

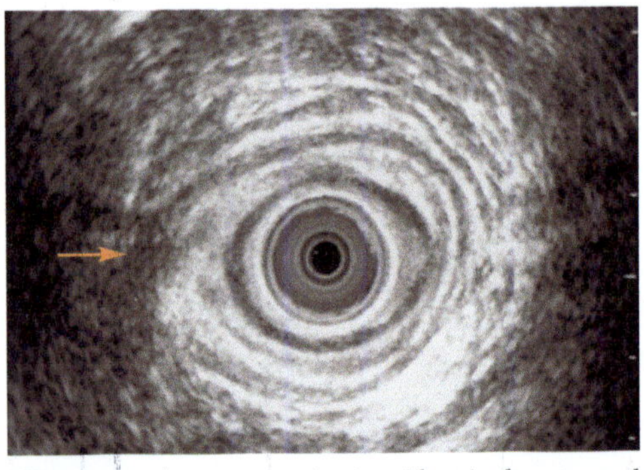

Fig. 16c. An abscess extension is evident in the retroanal space (*arrow*)

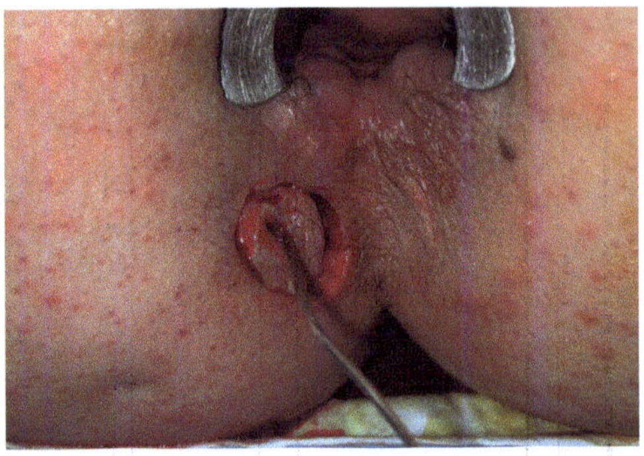

Fig. 16d. Commencement of the fistulectomy in this case, with a probe inserted into the external opening of the fistula

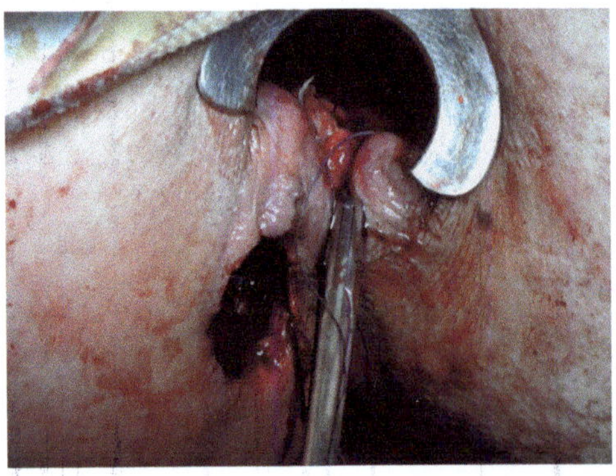

Fig. 16e. A rectal advancement flap was used here and sutured to the subcutaneous portion of the external anal sphincter. The ischiorectal abscess and the trans-sphincteric fistula have been excised

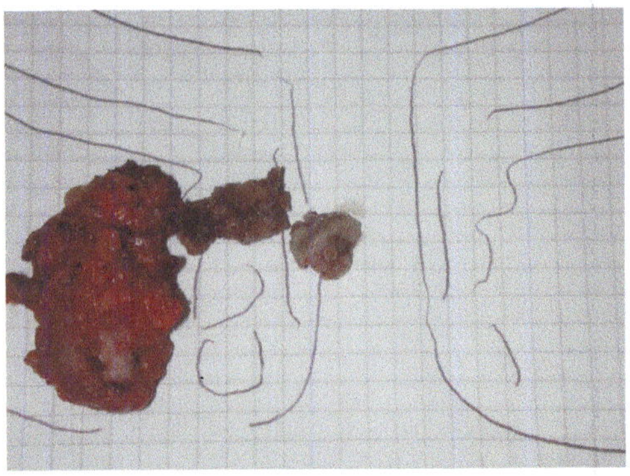

Fig. 16f. Specimen (i.e. the ischiorectal abscess and trans-sphincteric fistula (en bloc) and the retroanal abscess alongside an operative anorectal diagram. This approach is used by one of the authors (MP) as an operative teaching tool

Horseshoe Fistula

A 57 year-old man presented with perianal swelling, fever and malaise 3 years after a stapled hemorrhoidopexy followed by reintervention due to severe post-operative bleeding.

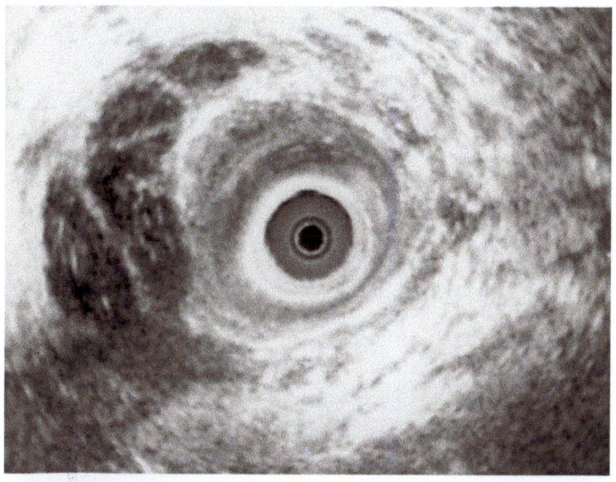

Fig. 17a. Endoanal ultrasound: a horseshoe posterior abscess is detected involving both intersphincteric and retroanal spaces

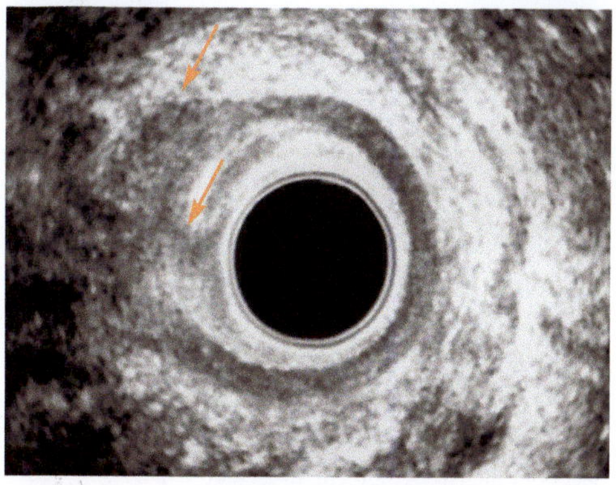

Fig. 17b. Endoanal ultrasound: posterior trans-sphincteric fistula and deep retroanal abscess (*arrow*)

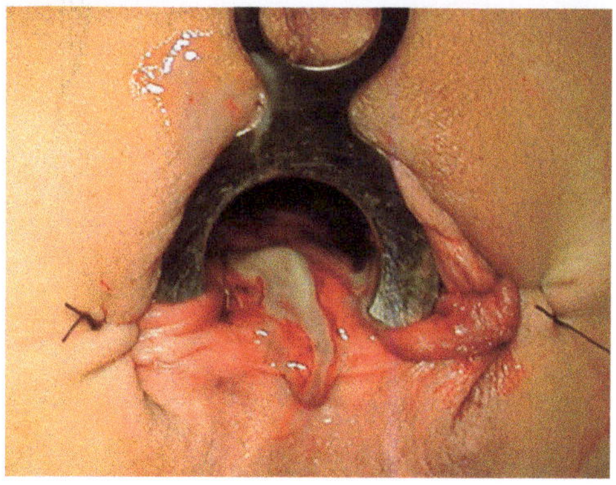

Fig. 17c. Operative field, patient in lithotomy position. Pus discharge through the posterior anal crypt

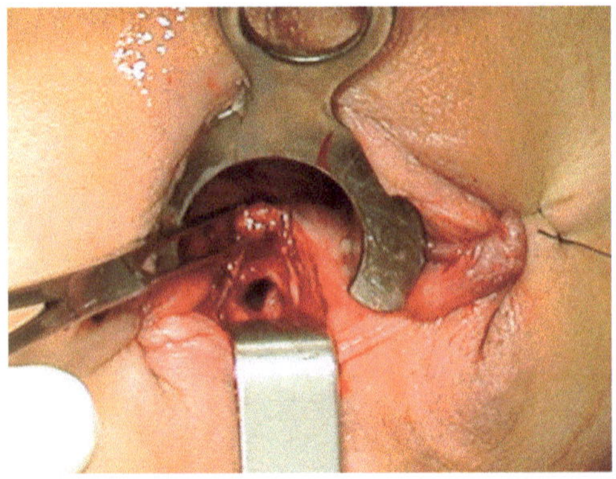

Fig. 17d. The posterior deep retroanal space is entered and drained

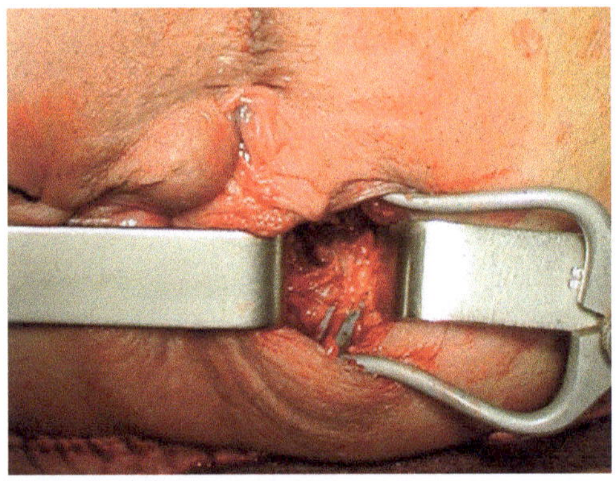

Fig. 17e. The left ischiorectal fossa is entered and drained. A fistulectomy had been carried out

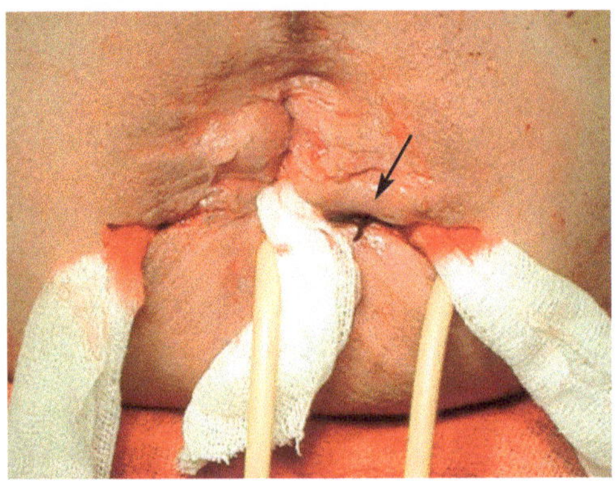

Fig. 17f. Final view of the operative field showing the retroanal opening filled with gauze and the two counter-incisions aimed at draining the ischiorectal fossae. Both the left ischiorectal fossa and deep retroanal space are drained by means of two Foley catheters. A draining seton has been inserted around the external sphincter (*arrow*)

Rectovaginal Fistula

Ano (or recto-) vaginal fistula may present as part of destructive perirectal sepsis and its preoperative recognition (sometimes in the face of minimal symptoms) may govern the surgical approach (transperineal versus endoanal). The only available study comparing endoanal sonography with endoanal MR imaging showed equivalent sensitivity and positive predictive value in the detection of rectovaginal fistulae [16].

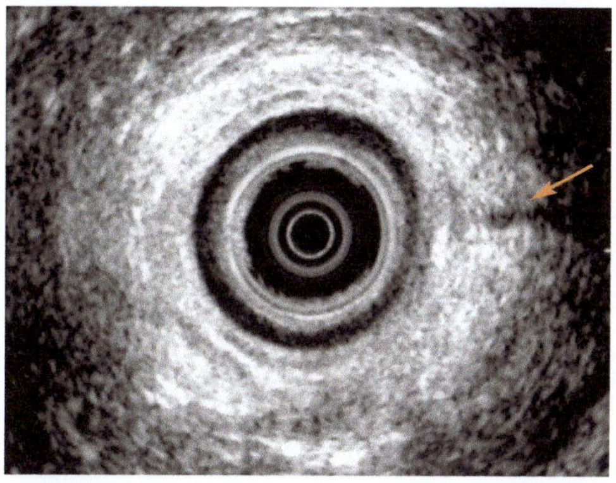

Fig. 18a. Rectovaginal fistula as shown by a hypoechoic track (*arrow*)

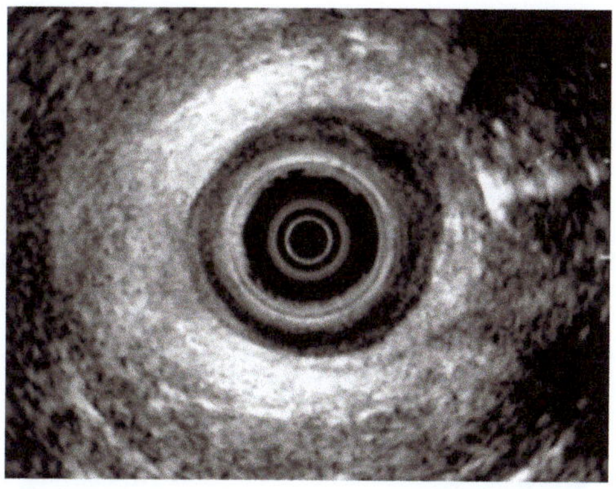

Fig. 18b. Hydrogen peroxide enhancement of the same patient leads to a readily recognizable hyperechoic effect

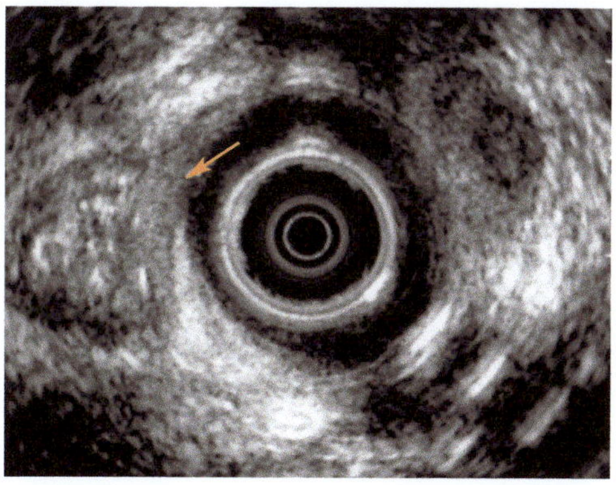

Fig. 18c. Transvaginal sonography of the same case (*arrow*)

Pouch-Cutaneous Fistula

A 46 year-old female patient had been submitted, 4 years previously, to a restorative proctocolectomy for an ulcerative colitis. She did well during these 4 years but then suddenly developed a pouch-cutaneous fistula with multiple external openings in the right thigh, fever and purulent discharge through the anus.

She had a laparotomy and diverting ileostomy performed but during the postoperative period the spur retracted, thus allowing distal passage of intestinal content. The patient presented with pouchitis, malaise and signs of local sepsis.

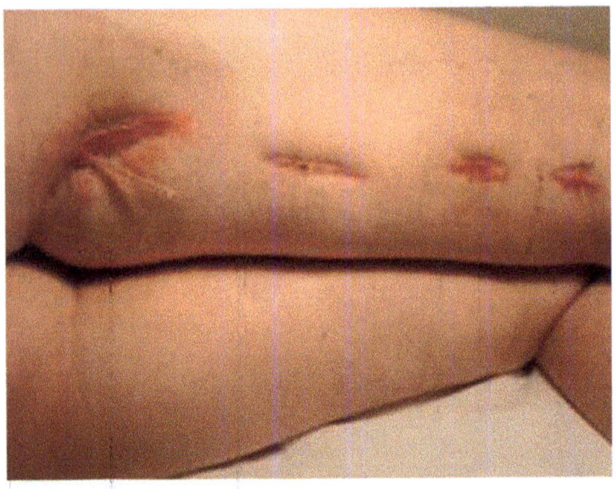

Fig. 19a. Clinical examination: multiple external openings in the right thigh from the popliteal fossa to the gluteal region

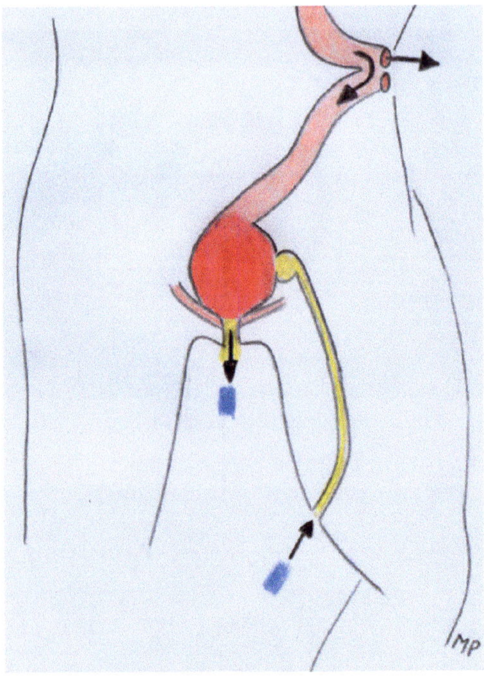

Fig. 19b. Methylene blue was injected in the cutaneous orifice showing a communication with the ileal reservoir, as illustrated in this diagram

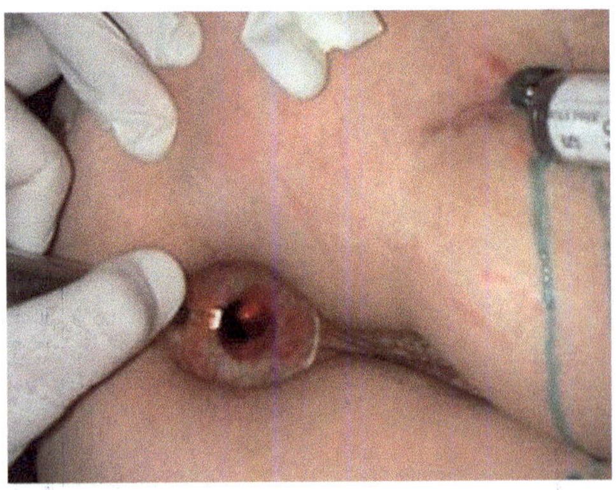

Fig. 19c. Endoscopic view of the pouch shows the methylene blue previously injected in the cutaneous orifice

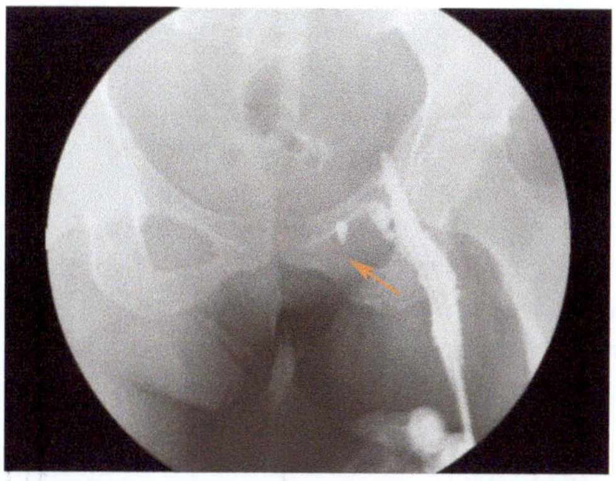

Fig. 19d. Fistulogram clearly shows a communication with the pouch through a perineal cavity (*arrow*)

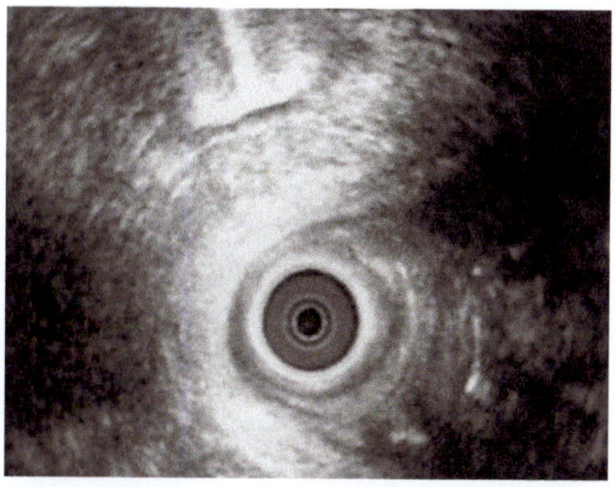

Fig. 19e. Anal ultrasound. A hyperechoic area highlighted by enhanced peroxide hydrogen injected through the external cutaneous orifice, is located above the puborectalis sling in the supralevator space. This area refers to the abscess cavity close to the ileal pouch

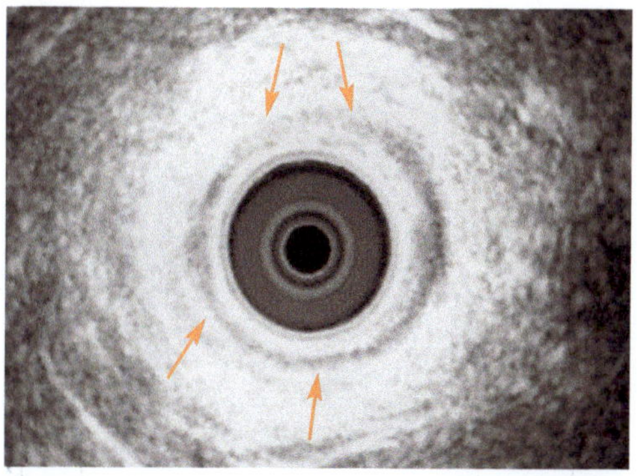

Fig. 19f. Anal ultrasound showing a diffused irregular internal sphincter (hypoechoic ring) with multiple defects (*arrows*) which may be related to the sphincter stretch during the transanal procedure of the restorative proctocolectomy. The hyperechoic ring of the external sphincter is intact as the patient is nulliparous

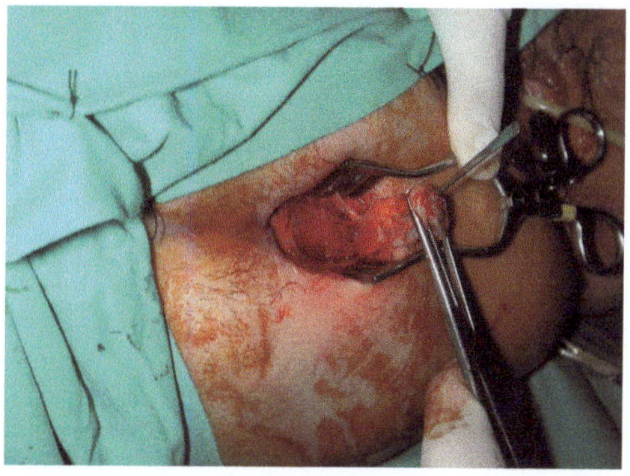

Fig. 19g. Transperineal phase of the operation: a probe inserted in the gluteal opening of the fistulous track shows the excision of the fistulous tract

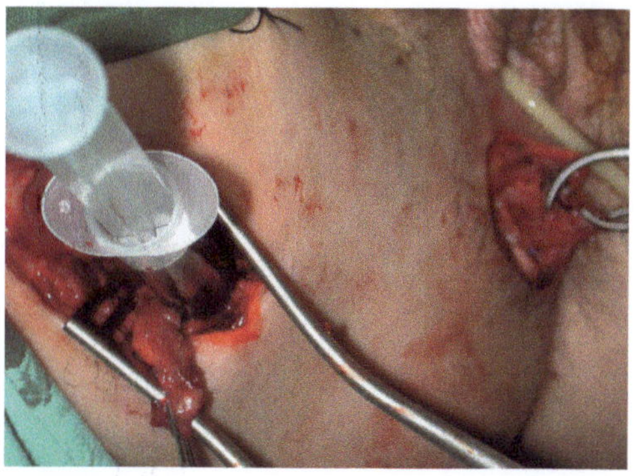

Fig. 19h. Injection of methylene blue into the gluteal external opening

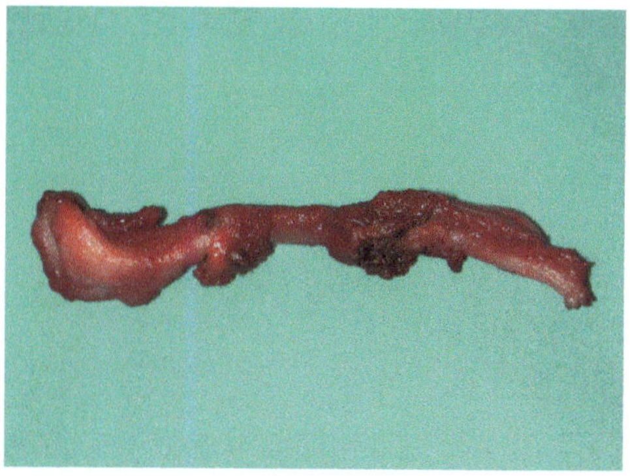

Fig. 19i. Surgical specimen of the excised fistulous track

Crohn's Disease

Perianal Crohn's disease provides at times a bewildering array of pathology with aberrantly located complex and deep fissures, complicated abscesses, fistulae and sinuses and endoanal stricturing. On occasion endoanal technology is impossible to utilize because of prior surgical induration or rectal stenosis occasioned by active disease, preventing deployment of the endorectal assembly. In some of these cases, it is advisable to more routinely use preoperative MRI or, where this is not available, transperineal sonography. The latter is more difficult to interpret but may have the advantage of being able to trace the course of distant sinuses and the disposition of rectovaginal fistulae. Serial imaging is particularly advantageous in patients being primarily treated with in-dwelling setons under Infliximab therapy. Endoanal ultrasound has the added value of defining the presence of destructive damage (or the effects of prior surgery) to the sphincters and the presence of anterior and/or posterior horseshoeing of sepsis in the indurated anal canal which is clinically difficult to evaluate.

Perianal Abscess

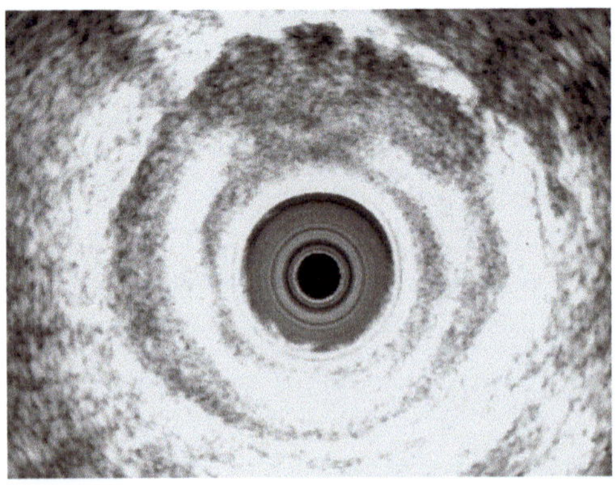

Fig. 20a. A right intersphincteric abscess in a multiply operated Crohn's patient

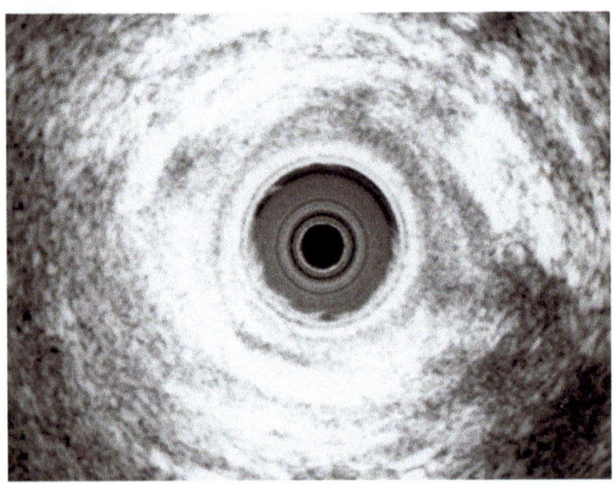

Fig. 20b. Perianal abscess extent on different level sectioning of the anal canal

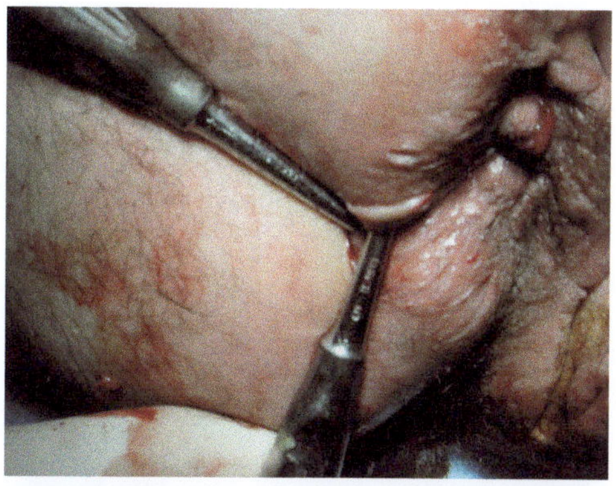

Fig. 20c. Drainage of the abscess in this case

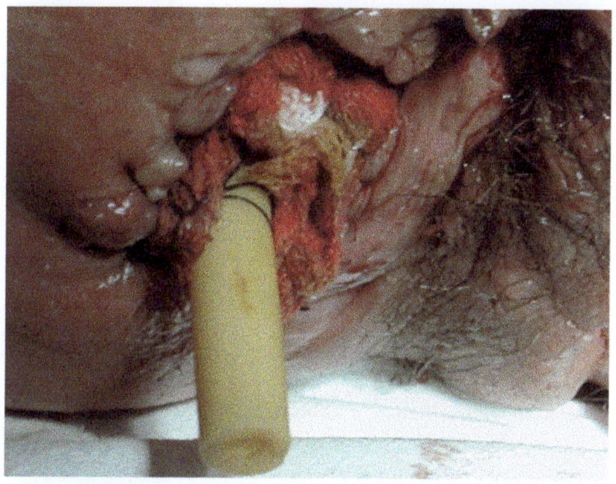

Fig. 20d. End of operation with insertion of a Petzer catheter

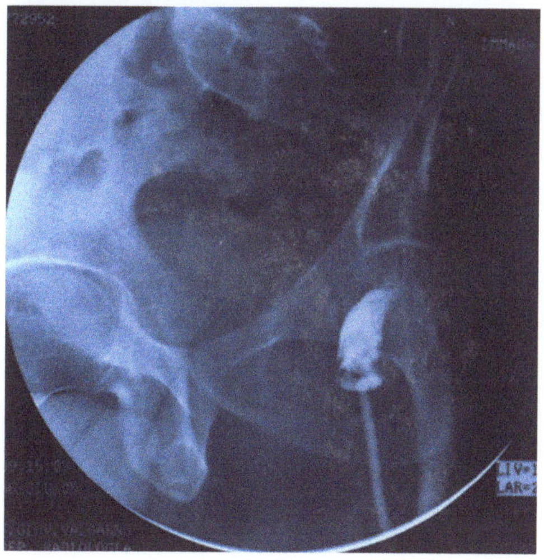

Fig. 20e. The catheter has been utilized to produce a postoperative sinogram to show the extent of the cavity and to direct the timing of catheter withdrawal

Recurrent Fistula

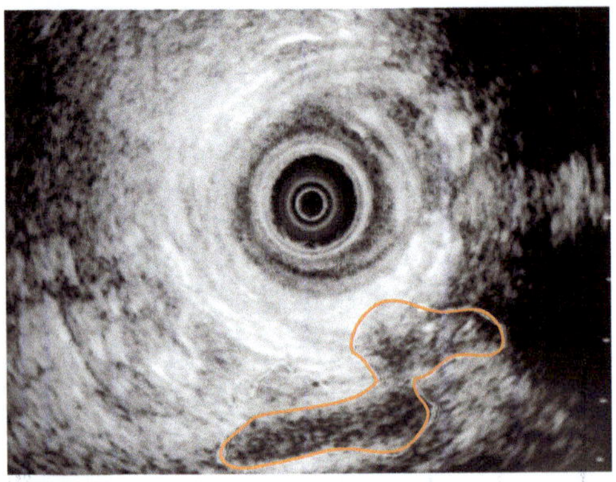

Fig. 21a. Left ischiorectal abscess (*marked*)

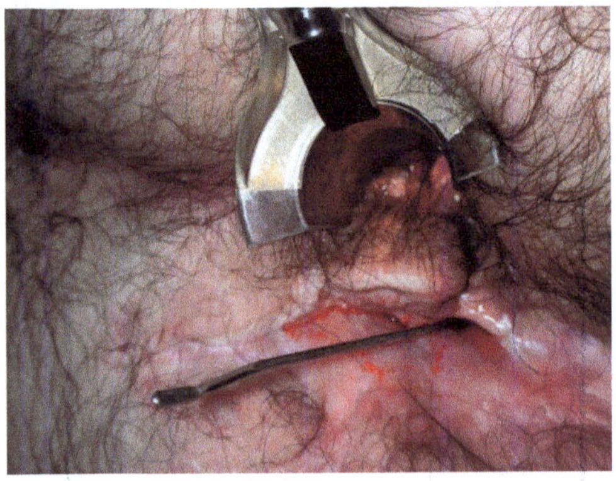

Fig. 21b. Fistula probing in the same patient. No communication with the anal canal is found

Fecal Incontinence

Endoanal ultrasonography has revolutionized the surgical diagnosis and management of patients presenting with fecal incontinence, replacing electromyographic sphincter mapping. The vast majority of patients present after complicated vaginal deliveries where there has been extended labor, episiotomy, forceps or vacuum extraction or associated large birth weight, [17] although there is still controversy over what represents the true incidence of anterior external anal sphincter defects [18]. This caveat aside, sonographic studies have correlated with intraoperative findings, [19] outcome and specific quality of life parametric analyses, with controversy still remaining concerning the prognostic significance of associated unilateral or bilateral pudendal neuropathy, [20] the initial algorithmic role of preliminary biofeedback therapy and the presence of heterogeneous internal anal sphincter defects [21]. Three-dimensional endoanal sonography has further demonstrated a correlation between the angle of the external anal sphincter defect and its coronal length, [22] implying that operative success of sphincteroplasty is dependent upon the coronal adequacy of the repair. Similar studies using endoanal MR imaging have further suggested that inherent external anal sphincter atrophy is quantifiable and also affects the functional outcome of repair even in experienced hands [23].

Obstetric Trauma

Multivariate analyses have shown that there are several prognostic factors in complicated delivery which are more likely to result in damage to both the anal sphincters; most notably, assisted delivery (either with forceps or vacuum extraction), the utilization of episiotomy and relative cephalopelvic disproportion. Such findings have been confirmed on prospective analysis. Endoanal ultrasonography has proven invaluable in the detection of both symptomatic and asymptomatic sphincter tears as well as guiding the use of initial biofeedback therapies, although there remains some controversy about the exact extent of the problem and the potential that endosonography has overcalled the incidence of significant anteriorly disposed sphincter defects [18, 24-29].

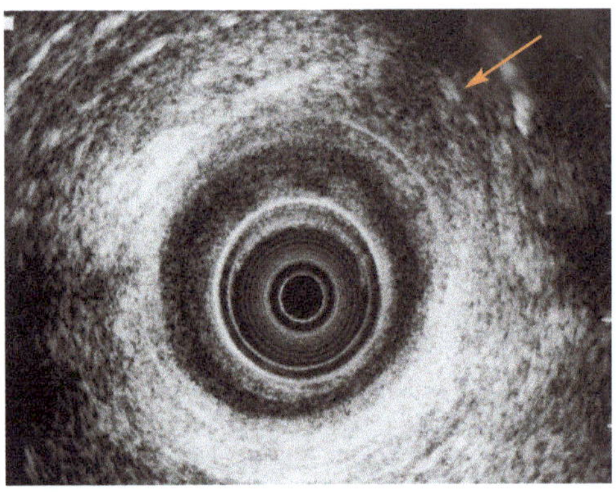

Fig. 22. A multiparous female patient presenting with fecal incontinence due to an antero-right lateral defect of the external anal sphincter (*arrow*)

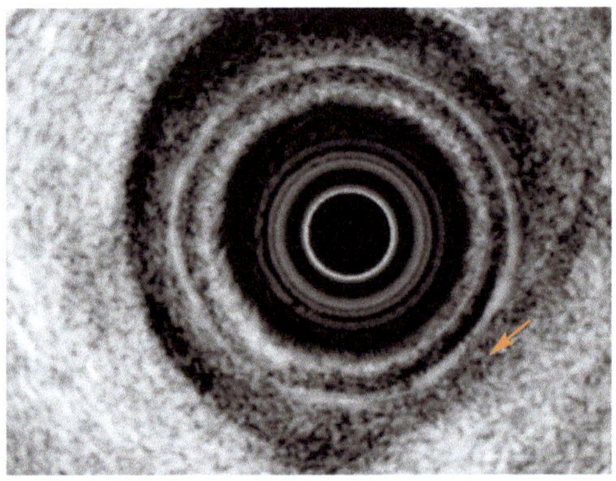

Fig. 23. Obstetric trauma mainly involving the internal anal sphincter (*arrow*): the scar has a hyperechoic appearance

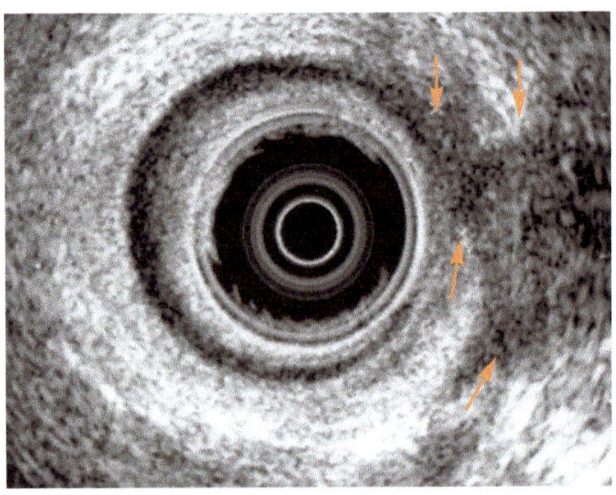

Fig. 24a. In this case there is a combined internal and external anal sphincter defect anteriorly (*arrows*)

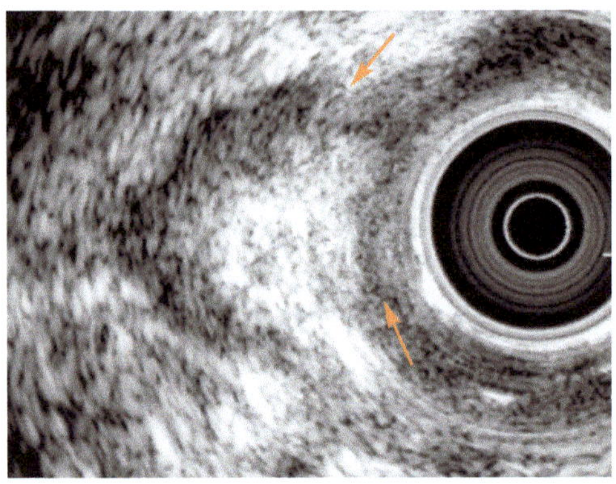

Fig. 24b. Transvaginal ultrasound of the same patient (*arrows*)

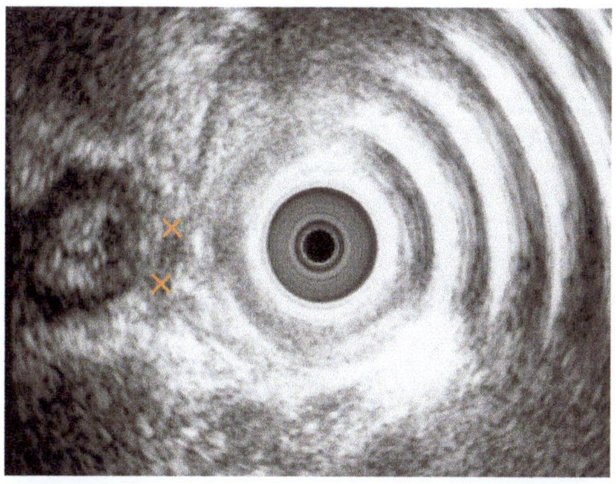

Fig. 25a. Transvaginal sonography showing an anterior defect of the external anal sphincter in a multiparous patient (*markers*)

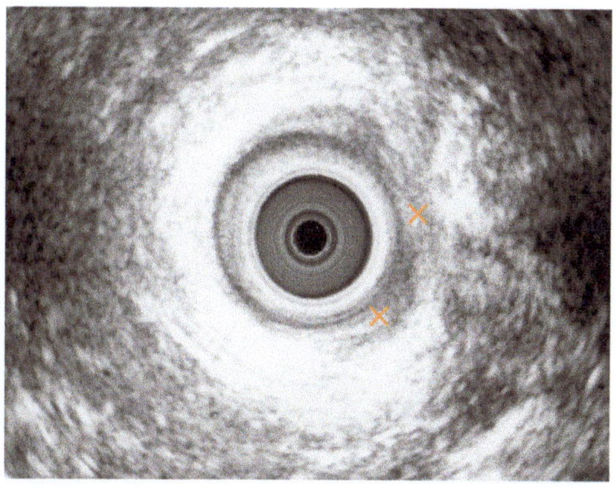

Fig. 25b. Endoanal ultrasound of the same patient showing the anterior muscle defect (*markers*)

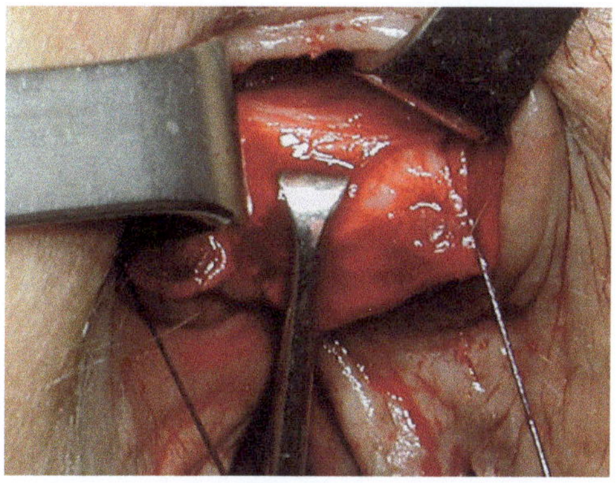

Fig. 25c. An anterior sphincter plication was performed

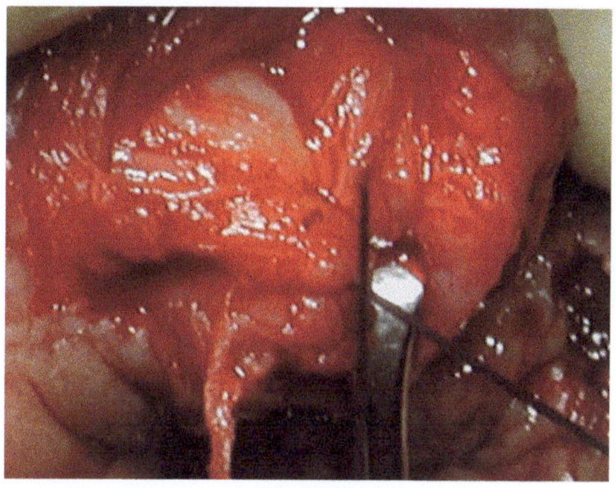

Fig. 25d. Completion of the plication

Following STARR Procedure

More recently, bulking agents have been used in an attempt to treat passive incontinence following internal anal sphincter damage [30, 31]. These agents have proved more efficient than internal anal sphincter plication and have included the utilization of silicone, [32] collagen [33] and autologous fat [34]. Their long term effects and exact indications appear unclear at present although endoanal sonography may be used for their real-time placement. The STARR double-stapled rectal resection procedure performed for rectocele and internal mucosal prolapse along with some of the newer hemorrhoid surgeries including Ligasure hemorrhoidectomy, Doppler-guided hemorrhoid artery ligation and stapled hemorrhoidopexy, make no attempt to separate the internal anal sphincter from the hemorrhoidal complex. In this event, particularly where there is significant pre-existing hemorrhoidal prolapse, there is the potential for significant internal sphincter damage; an effect which is more typically avoided in open hemorrhoidectomy where a deliberate attempt is made to separate the mucosal complex from the sphincter muscle.

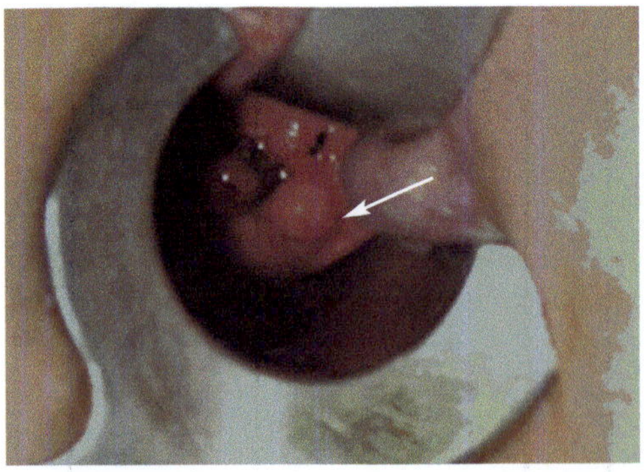

Fig. 26a. Rubber band ligation of recurrent rectal internal mucosa prolapse after the STARR operation for obstructed defecation. The *arrow* shows a small polypoid pyogenic granuloma around one of the staples

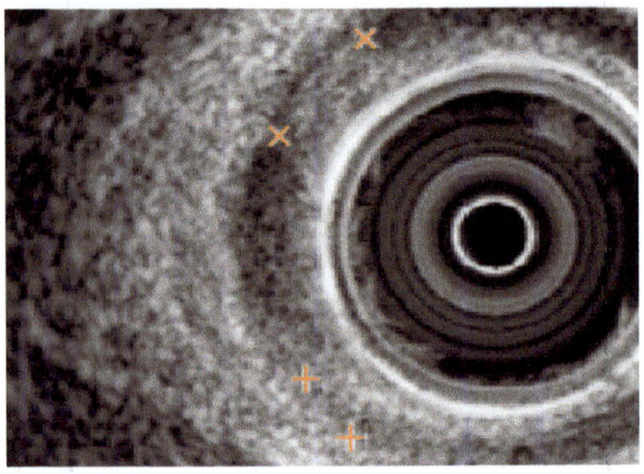

Fig. 26b. Anal US showing two interruptions of the internal anal sphincter (*markers*)

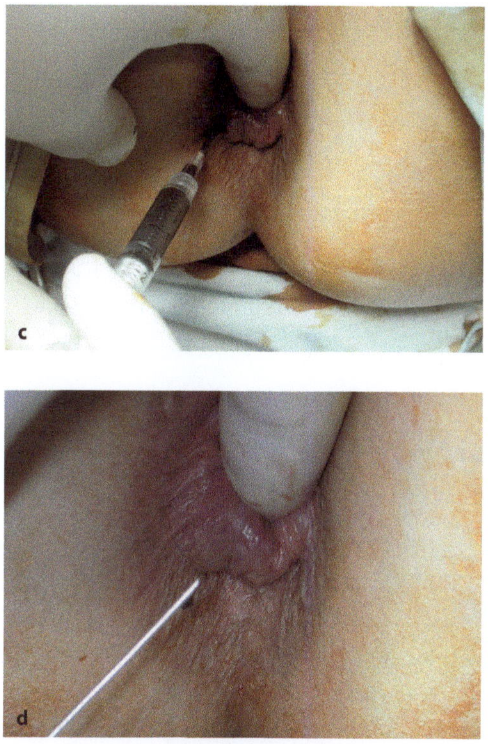

Fig. 26c, d. The patient, a 47 year-old multiparous female, complained of minor daily fecal soiling. In this case injection of the bulking agent Durasphere® was performed under local anesthetic

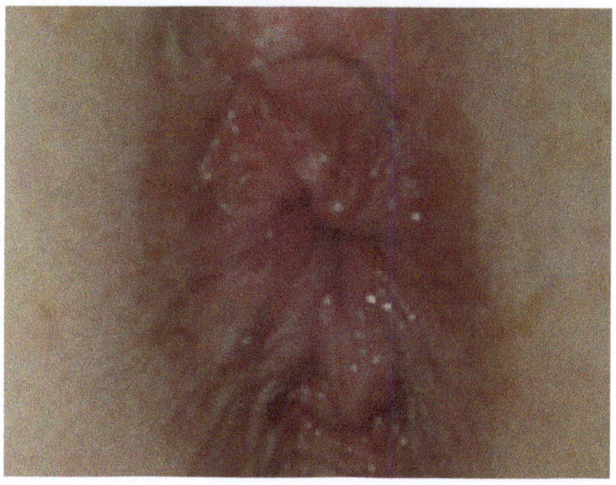

Fig. 26e. The appearance of the 'closed anus' following Durasphere® injection

Fecal incontinence and Recurrent Rectal Prolapse

A multiparous 73 year-old woman who suffered from urinary incontinence related to a cystocoele, and obstructed defecation with fecal incontinence, complained of a prolapsing external bulk on straining. She underwent a defecography that showed a mild rectocele and a rectal mucosal prolapse, therefore a STARR (Stapled trans anal rectal resection) procedure and a cystopexy were undertaken. The patient had an early recurrence of both constipation and rectal prolapse, moreover after surgery she complained of very painful perineal heaviness and tenesmus. The patient was then visited at our Unit. At clinical examination a patulous anus was evident and a full thickness rectal prolapse protruded after straining in the squatting position. An anal endosonography was performed and then a new surgical procedure was planned.

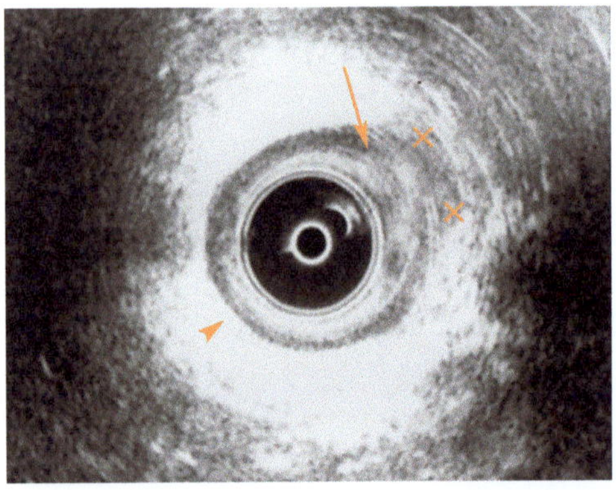

Fig. 27a. Anal ultrasound shows an internal mucosal prolapse, prevalently anterior (*arrow*). The shape of the hypoechoic ring of the internal sphincter is irregular posteriorly, possibly due to surgical damage (*arrowhead*). The sphincter is also thin anteriorly partly covered by the mucosal prolapse and possibly due to obstetric damage because of vaginal deliveries. More evident sphincter damage, most probably related to vaginal deliveries, is seen in the deep part of the external sphincter (*markers*)

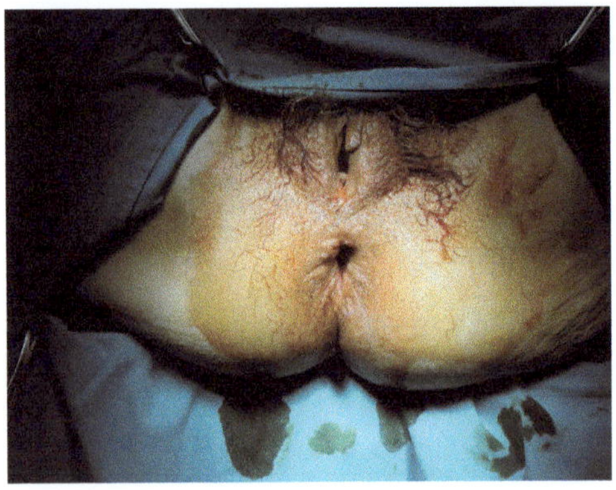

Fig. 27b. Prior to reintervention, at clinical examination, a patulous anus was evident

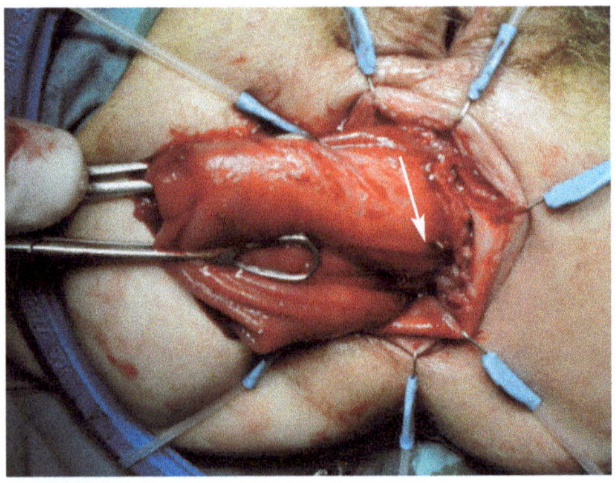

Fig. 27c. Operative field: a full thickness external prolapse, 8 cm in size, is pulled out. A Lonestar retractor has been positioned and allows detection of a retained staple from the previous surgical procedure (*arrow*)

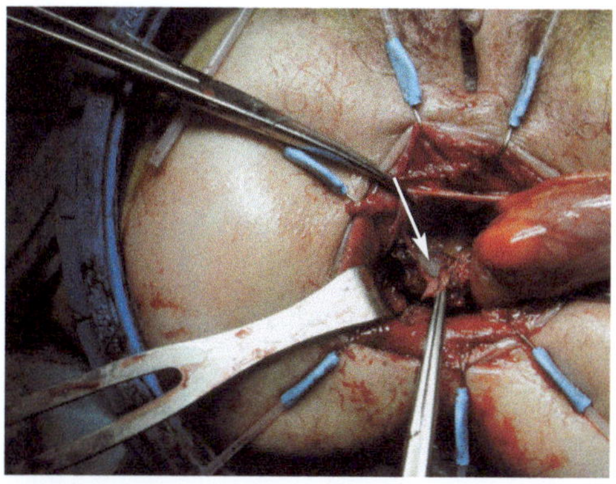

Fig. 27d. The first step of the Altemeier procedure is completed: the prolapsed peritoneal pouch has been opened revealing an enterocele (*arrow*)

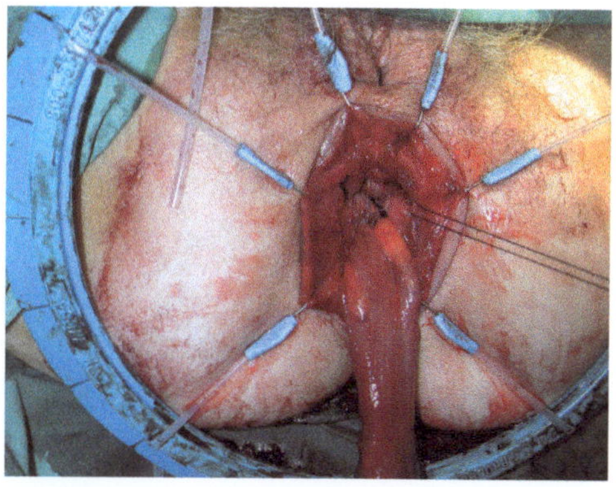

Fig. 27e. The anterior levatorplasty is carried out

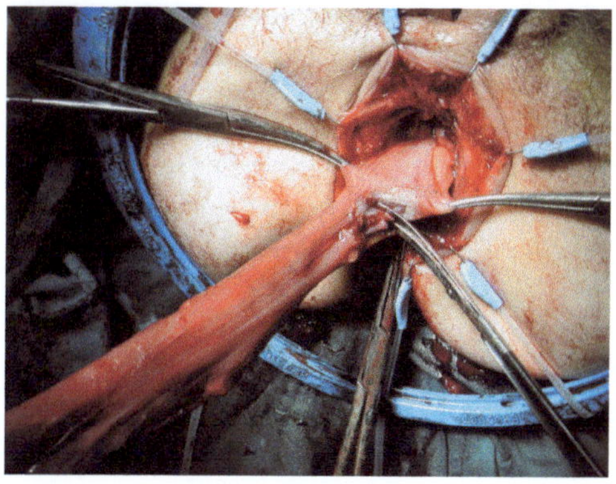

Fig. 27f. The rectum is being resected

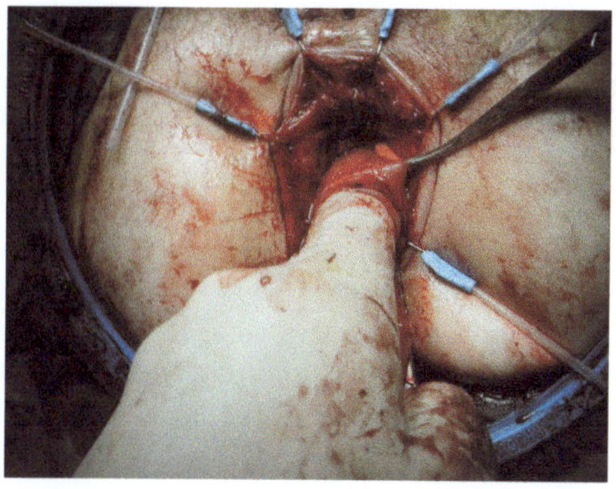

Fig. 27g. The colon is ready for the colo-anal anastomosis

Postsurgical Miscellanea

Post-surgical endoanal sonograms may be difficult to interpret, particularly where distinction is to be made between postoperative scarring and recrudescent sepsis [35]. Here images may be supplemented by Gadolinium-enhanced MR imaging (either surface or endoanal MR fistulography) which will assist in defining active collections and tracks [36, 37]. The newer techniques of more limited hemorrhoidectomy and hemorrhoidopexy as well as the STARR endoanal stapled procedure for rectocele exclusion may inadvertently injure the IAS, resulting in heterogenous sphincter injury [38].

Postoperative Fibrosis and Abscess

Postoperative fibrosis may be difficult to separate from recrudescent sepsis, where there is in endorectal ultrasound no essential difference between burnt out and persistent inflammation. This is of importance in the multiply reoperated case (particularly when there is underlying perianal Crohn's disease) and where there is so much induration that clinical examination is unreliable. Here too, endoanal ultrasonography can overcall relatively large intersphincteric collections as trans-sphincteric in nature because of acoustic shadowing behind the collection and this may place more sphincter at risk if the ultrasound is solely relied upon for surgical drainage. In these cases, again, MRI with Gadolinium enhancement is more desirable since it will more adequately define active from quiescent sepsis. Serial ultrasonography in such patients assessing for changes within the intersphincteric space may prove useful.

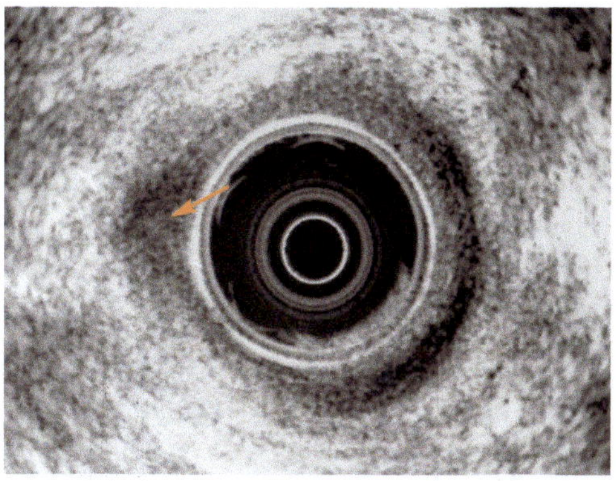

Fig. 28. A mixed echogenicity lesion is evident following a posterior anal fistulectomy (*arrow*)

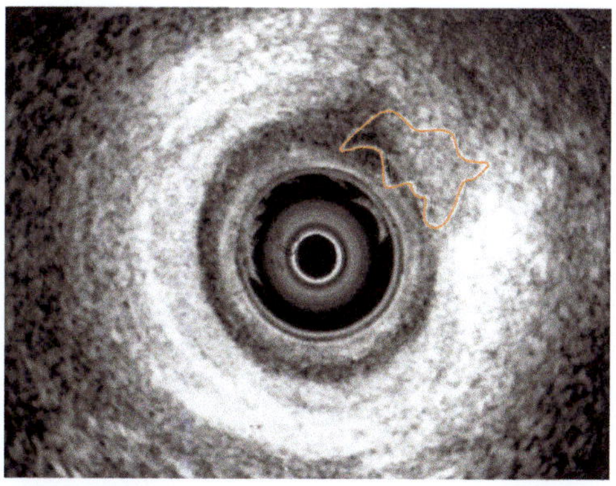

Fig. 29. Following hemorrhoidectomy. A lesion of the internal anal sphincter is evident with fibrosis of the intersphincteric plane (*marked*)

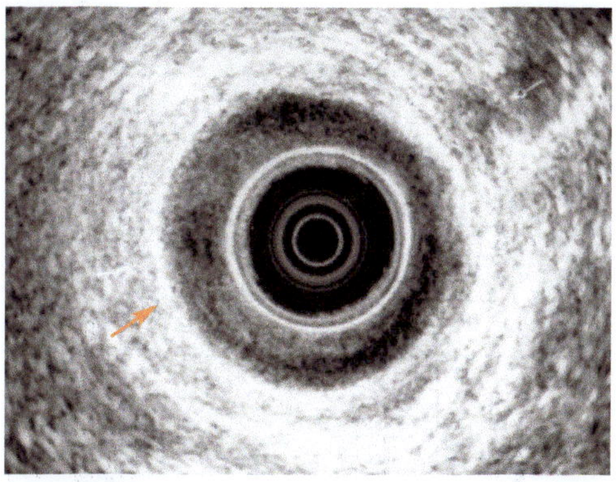

Fig. 30. The internal anal sphincter is involved by postoperative fibrosis and partially covered by a rectal internal mucosal prolapse posteriorly (*arrow*)

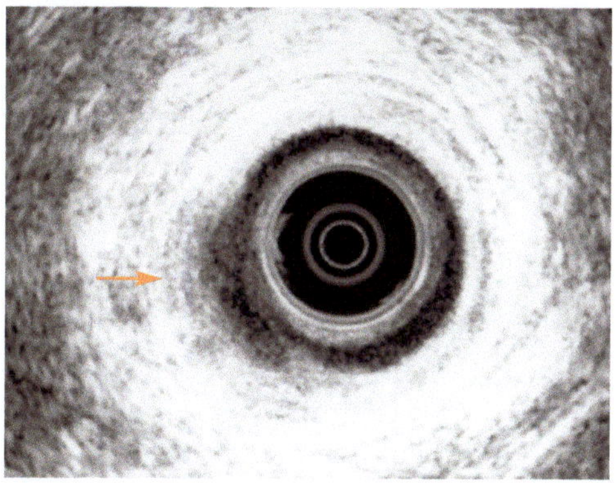

Fig. 31. Early postoperative intersphincteric fibrosis (*arrow*)

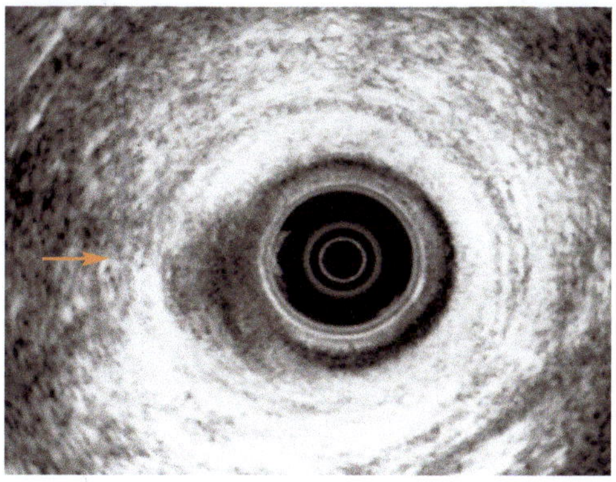

Fig. 32. Postoperative inter-and-perisphincteric fibrosis (*arrow*)

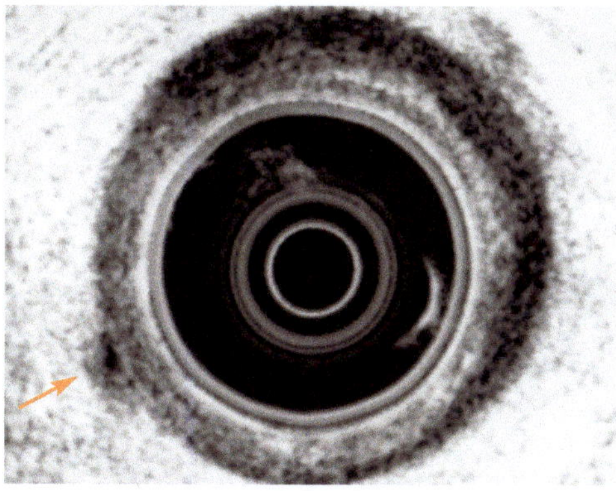

Fig. 33. Posterior intersphincteric chronic abscess post-hemorrhoidectomy (*arrow*)

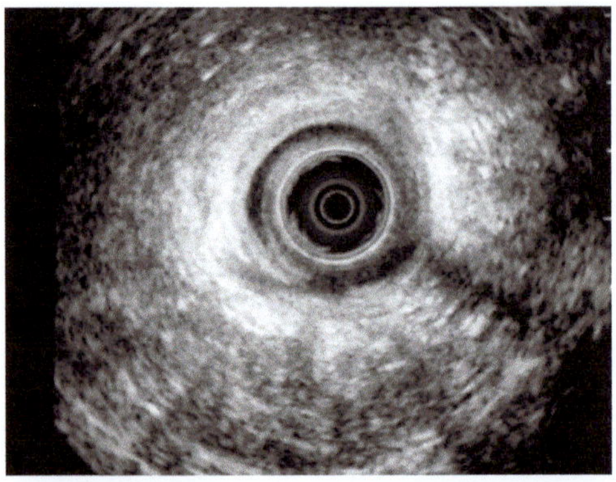

Fig. 34. Left anterolateral postfistulectomy fibrosis mimicking fistula recurrence. Partial interruption of the internal sphincter is due to the surgical drainage of the intersphincteric plane and is a common finding

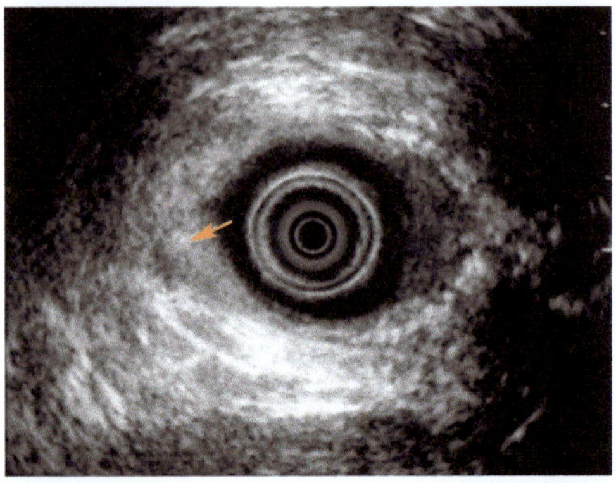

Fig. 35. A postanal chronic abscess is still evident after fistulectomy (*arrow*)

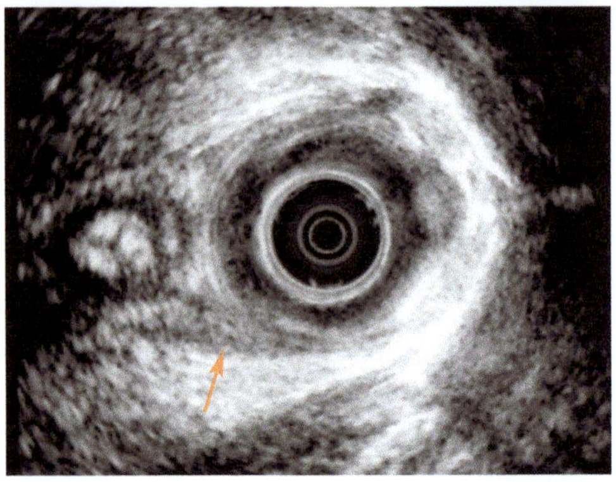

Fig. 36. Transvaginal postfistulectomy ultrasound showing a left lateral perianal mixed hyperechoic area (*arrow*) mimicking a recurrent abscess

Post Milligan-Morgan Hemorrhoidectomy, Stapled Hemorrhoidopexy and STARR

Many local anal anomalies are demonstrable following hemorrhoid surgery, including deep seated perirectal sepsis, inadvertent sphincter injury and staple line disruption [39-42]. Newer techniques such as Ligasure hemorrhoidectomy, Doppler-guided hemorrhoid artery ligation and PPH stapled hemorrhoidopexy make no specific attempt to separate the hemorrhoidal complex from the IAS, potentially rendering this sphincter muscle at greater risk than open techniques.

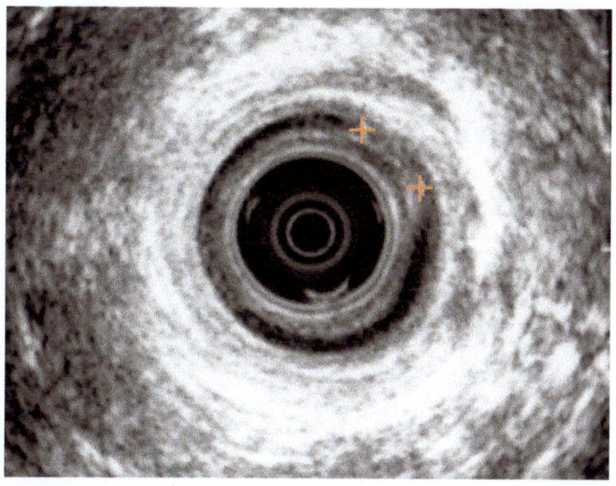

Fig. 37. Posthemorrhoidectomy injury to the internal sphincter (*markers*)

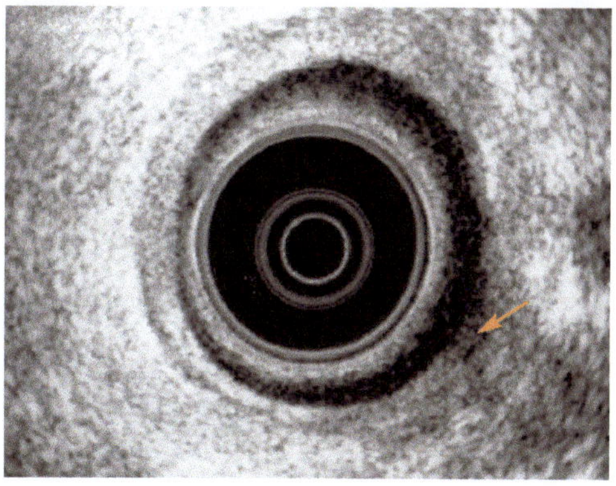

Fig. 38. Proctalgia secondary to an anterolateral postoperative chronic abscess (*arrow*)

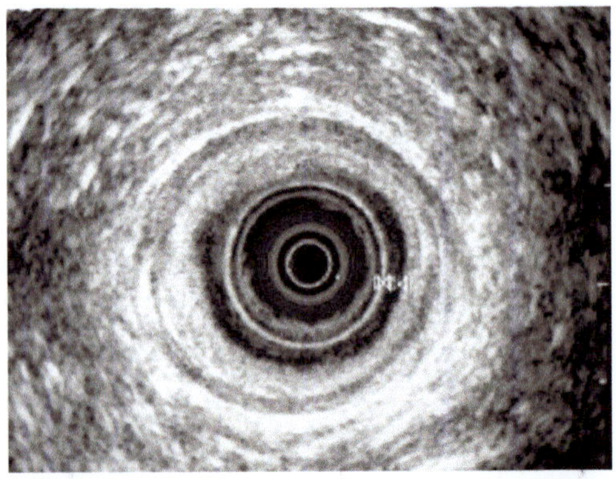

Fig. 39. Lower anal canal endoanal ultrasound. Postoperative internal sphincter's lesion due to concomitant anal stretch caused by the CAD anal dilator: the internal sphincter (hyperechoic ring) is thin and heterogeneously fragmented

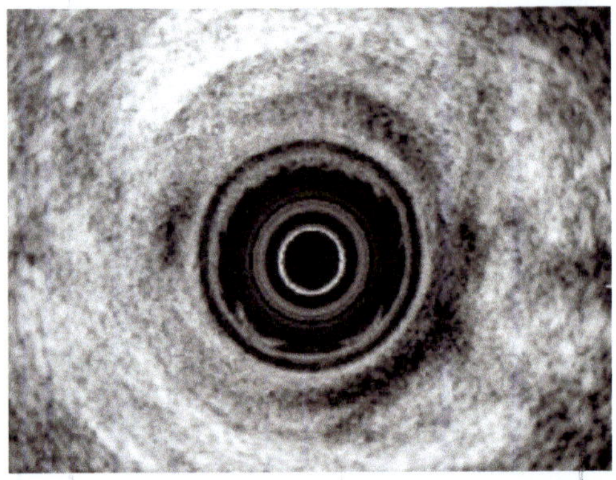

Fig. 40. In a similar case, the lower edge of the internal sphincter is interrupted. The patient has fecal soiling following stapled hemorrhoidopexy

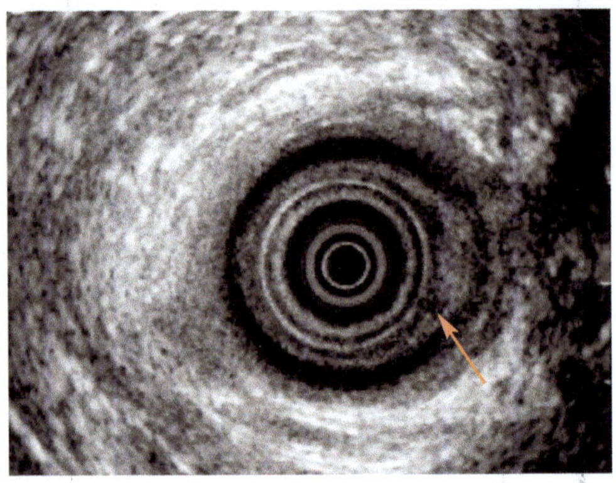

Fig. 41. Upper anal canal. Incontinence, proctalgia, rectocele and constipation followed a STARR double stapled transanal rectotomy. There is evidence of recurrent or residual anterior rectal internal mucosal prolapse (*arrow*)

Evacuatory Disorders

Enterocele and Rectal Intussusception

Enteroceles are more typically evident in patients following hysterectomy, particularly where coincident culposuspension is not performed [43-45]. Their diagnosis is essential in rectocele patients presenting with evacuatory difficulty since rectocele repair alone will be relatively unsuccessful. Enteroceles are traditionally diagnosed by extended defecography and more recently by dynamic magnetic resonance imaging, but may still be missed in 20% of cases [46]. More recently, dynamic transperineal ultrasonography has been successful in their diagnosis [47]. Recto-rectal and recto-anal intussusception, mainly diagnosed at defecography, may appear in normal subjects but also cause obstructed defecation and low rectal lesions [48].

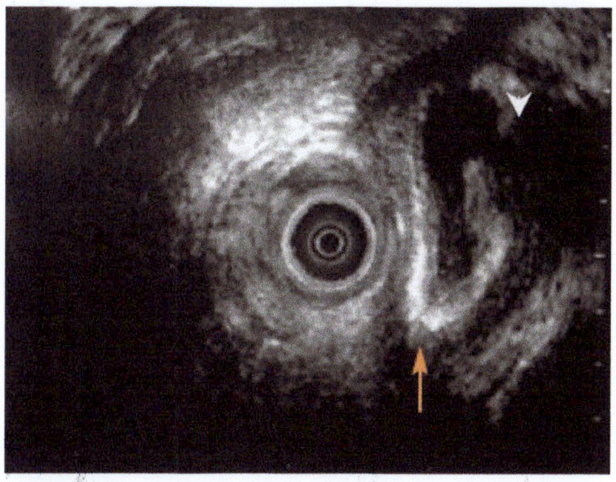

Fig. 42. Anterior descent of an intestinal loop (*arrow*) interposed between the rectum and vagina evident anteriorly (*arrowhead*)

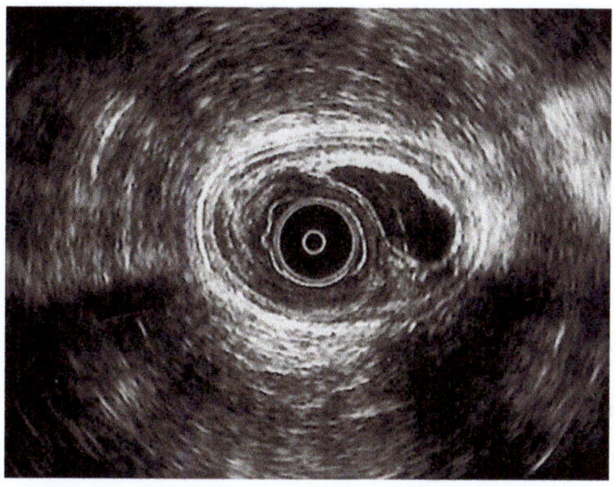

Fig. 43. Rectal internal intussusception in which a full thickness double layer is seen during straining

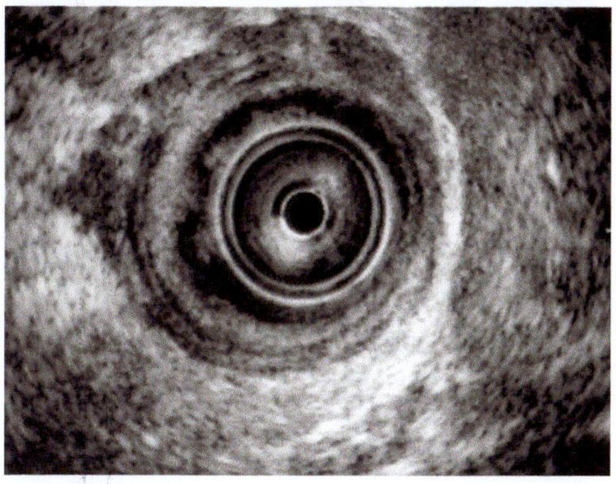

Fig. 44. Low rectal intussusception as evident by a double layer recognizable on endosonography

Solitary Rectal Ulcer Syndrome (SRUS)

SRUS is a comparatively uncommon cause of evacuatory discomfort, often associated with specific psychological traits, rectal digitation and chronic constipation. It is believed to be associated with rectoanal intussusception and may represent a forme fruste of full-thickness rectal prolapse since there is a variable response to resection rectopexy. It is often not ulcerative as such and may not on endoscopy be solitary, but is characterized by classical histological reorientation of the muscularis mucosae fibers into a vertical disposition [49].

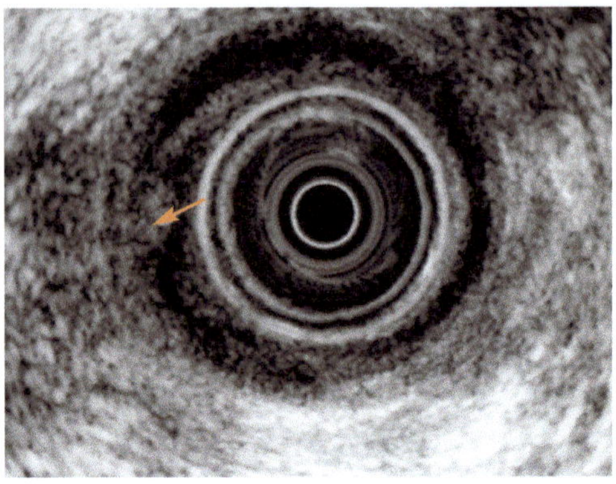

Fig. 45a. The *arrow* indicates the 'polypoid lesion' evident at the anorectal ring

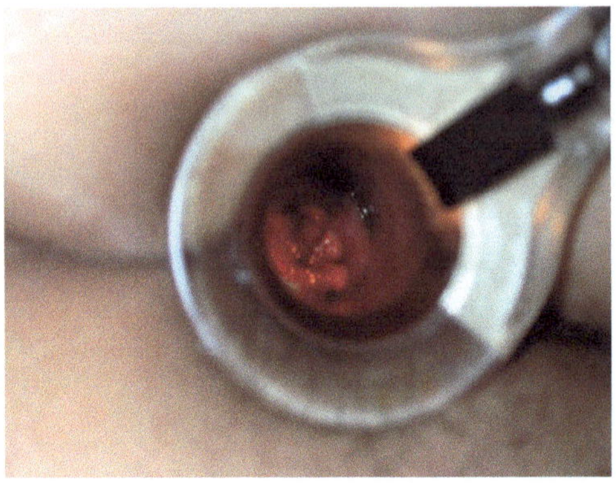

Fig. 45b. Proctoscopic view of the SRUS lesion at the level of the anorectal ring

Rectal Internal Mucosal Prolapse

Rectal internal mucosal prolapse may be proctoscopically graded depending upon the degree of descensus of the mucosa towards the anal verge [50]. It is typically associated with other pelvic floor disorders presenting with the symptom complex of evacuatory difficulty, most notably rectocele. Greater grades have been successfully treated with either stapled mucosal prolapsectomy [51], but long-term results has been found to be unsatisfactory in half of the patients following either manual or stapled prolapsectomy [52].

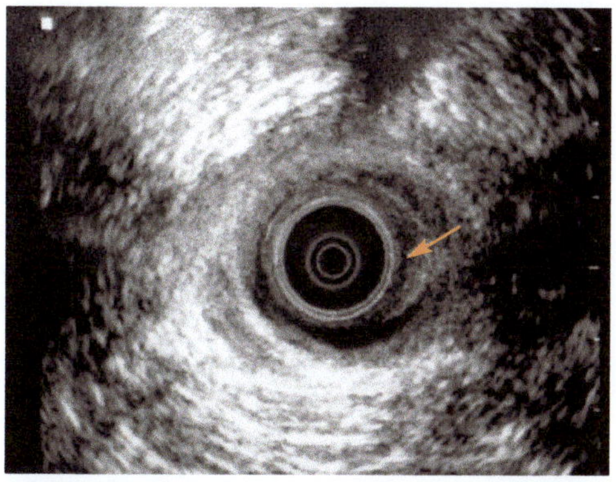

Fig. 46. Upper anal canal endoanal ultrasound. Anterior rectal internal mucosal prolapse is shown by the *arrow*

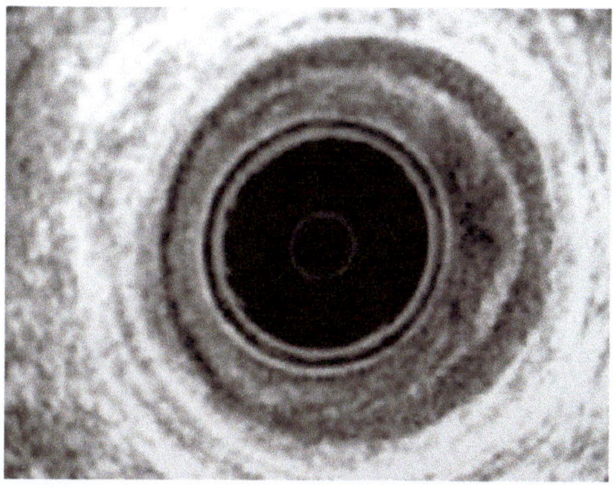

Fig. 47. Middle anal canal endoanal ultrasound (magnified view) showing circumferential rectal internal mucosal prolapse in front of the hypoechoic internal anal sphincter

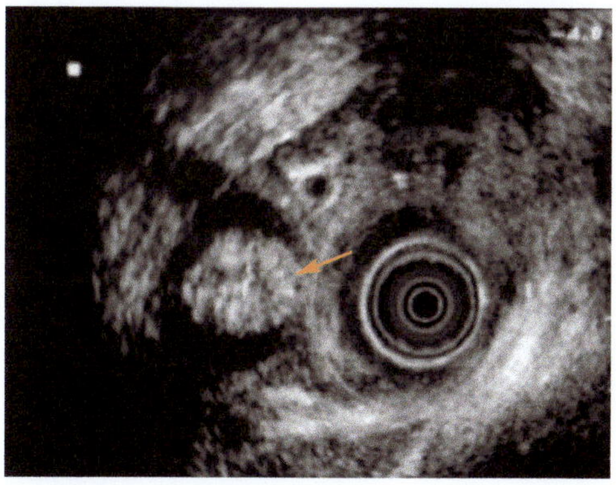

Fig. 48a. Transvaginal ultrasound performed at the level of the anorectal ring. The circle of the hypoechoic internal sphincter is thinner anteriorly (*arrow*) due to a muscle defect and to prolapsed rectal mucosa. The patient also had a rectocele

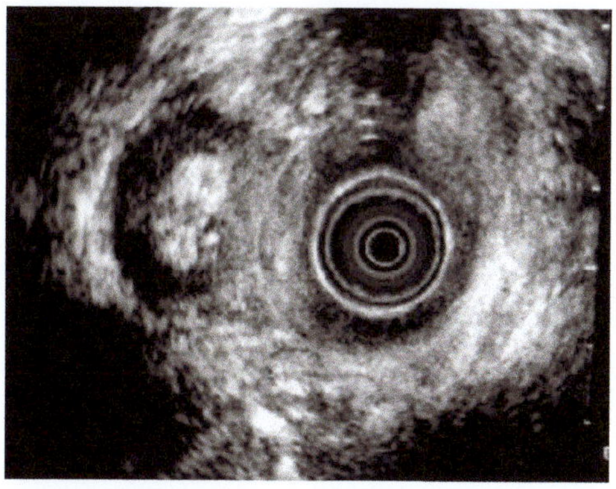

Fig. 48b. Transvaginal ultrasound in the middle anal canal, the internal sphincter defect is more evident

Anismus

Paradoxical puborectalis contraction (anismus) is difficult to diagnose, and is an important cause of evacuatory dysfunction where there is unexpected levator floor contraction during forced evacuation [53]. Its presence has been traditionally diagnosed by defecographic indentation of the puborectalis during straining, by difficulty of patient balloon evacuation (or elimination of a simulated fecal bolus) or by inversion of the normal rectoanal manometric pressure profile during forcible straining [54-56]. Its preoperative identification has been linked to a range of psychological dysfunctions which manifest as somatization disorders and its detection before surgery has in some series predicted for a worse functional outcome in patients operated upon for a range of surgically remediable disorders which manifest as defecation difficulty; most notably, rectocele, descending perineum syndrome, rectal prolapse, rectoanal intussusception and solitary rectal ulcer syndrome [57].

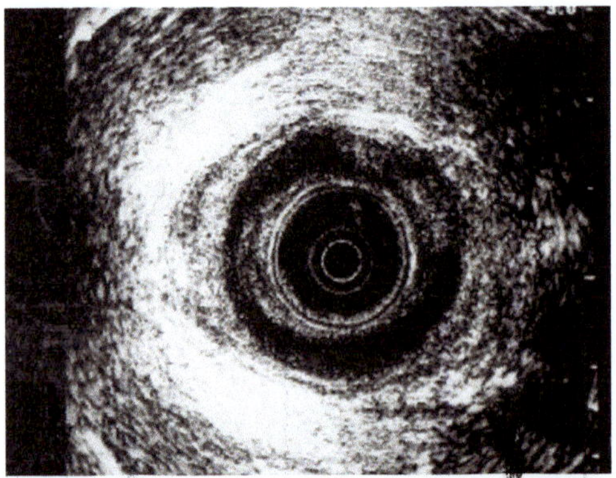

Fig. 49a. Upper anal canal endoanal ultrasound at rest. The puborectalis muscle is shown as a hyperechoic sling lying on its side

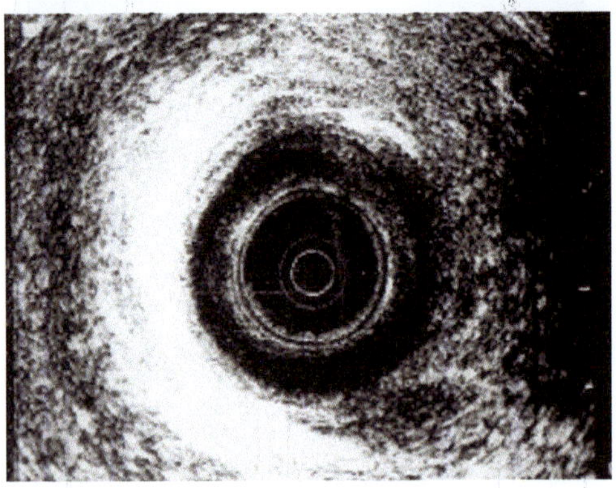

Fig. 49b. Paradoxical contraction of the puborectalis muscle on forcible straining in the same patient (Reproduced from [39])

Congenital Conditions

Rectal Duplication

Duplications of the alimentary tract are particularly uncommon, with rectal duplication itself representing only between 1-8% of all alimentary duplications [58] and rarely presenting in the adult [59]. These lesions can be cystic, tubular or fistulating, presenting with pain and prolapse or as complex perirectal sepsis. Most are retrorectal and are best excised in toto because of the potential for malignant transformation or for recurrent epithelial satellites, although very low lying or infected lesions may be treated by complete mucosectomy using either a transanal or posterior sagittal approach [60].

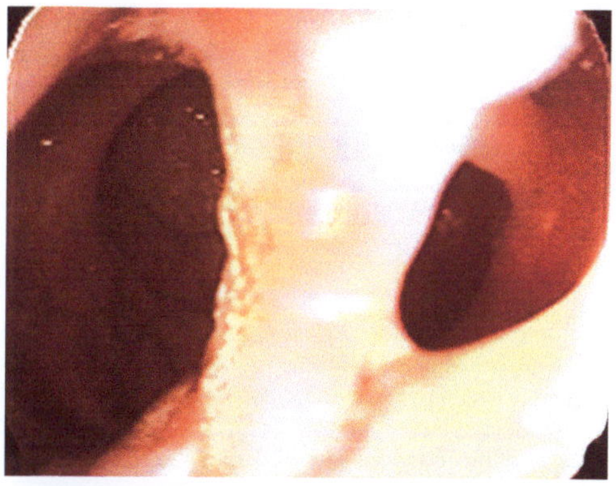

Fig. 50a. Endoscopic appearance of the rectal duplication

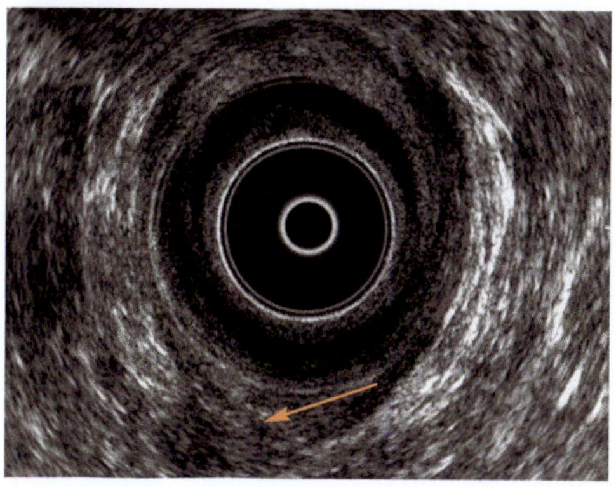

Fig. 50b. Endoanal ultrasound showing a trans-sphincteric hypoechoic mass (*arrow*) which was a rectal duplication cyst in a 43 year-old man who presented with perianal discomfort and incomplete evacuation. The duplication was treated by mucosectomy combined with a stapled division of the duplication bridge because of its close location to the lower intersphincteric plane. Patient in lithotomy position (Courtesy of A.P. Zbar)

Imperforate Anus Following Cut-Back Anoplasty

Both endoluminal and transperineal (vide infra) sonography may be used to assess imperforate anus although there is limited data available. This may be coupled by surface MR imaging to define the integrity of the levator plate which can be unilaterally or bilaterally deficient [61]. The advantages include the delineation of urinary fistulae in high anomalies and the status of the lower sphincters in low anomalies; most notably in vestibular anus and covered anus.

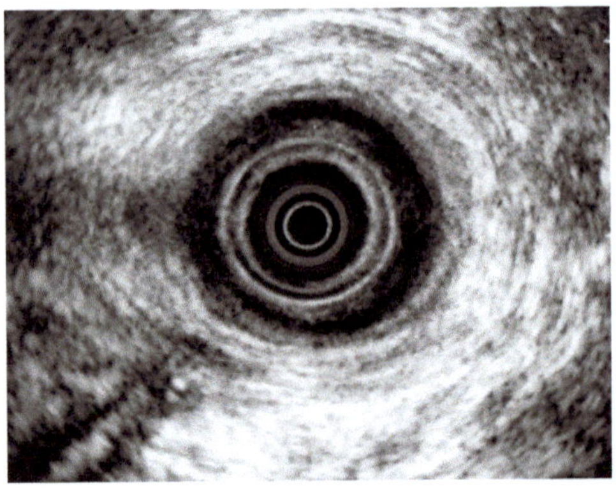

Fig. 51a. In this case, the endoluminal probe was introduced into the anteriorly disposed perineal sinus (i.e. the ectopic anal canal). The patient, 54 year-old, had previously undergone a cut- back anoplasty shortly after birth and presented with mild fecal incontinence and moderate soiling through the ectopic anal canal

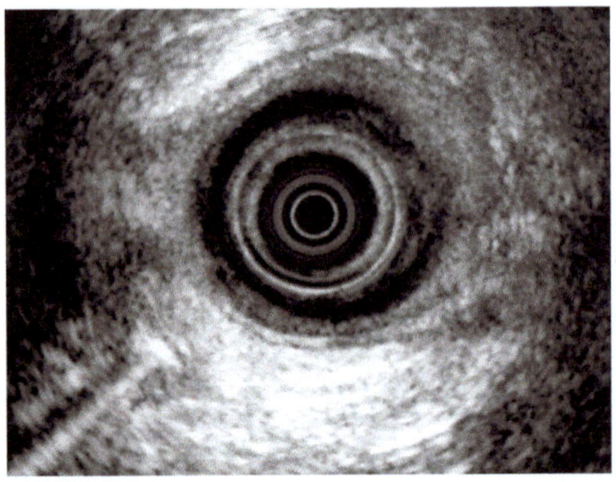

Fig. 51b. Injection of hydrogen peroxide through the eye of the probe. Both the internal and external anal sphincters are well formed

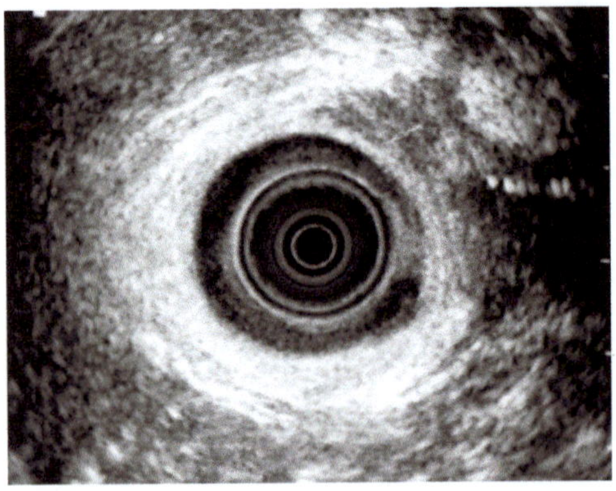

Fig. 51c. The intact internal anal sphincter is almost complete in this high anal canal view

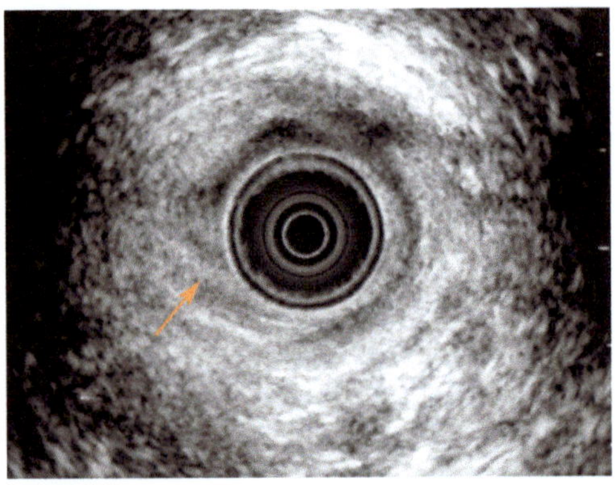

Fig. 51d. Other views show dyshomogeneity and interruption (*arrow*) of the internal anal sphincter which is the main contributing factor to this patient's passive incontinence

Anal Fissure

Incontinence has been variably reported following lateral internal anal sphincterotomy with considerable evidence to show that the extent of the sphincterotomy correlates with both postoperative functional outcome as well as specific quality of life [61-65]. This issue is complex since there may be concomitant inadvertent external anal sphincter damage in some cases and the effect of destructive postoperative deep seated perirectal sepsis. In some patients no significant demonstrable sphincter injury (beyond localized internal anal sphincterotomy) is detected and here there may be relatively subtle variations in the character and parameters of the rectoanal inhibitory reflex (an internal anal sphincter function) as well as constitutive variations in external anal sphincter overlap of the termination of the internal anal sphincter whereby internal sphincterotomy could render the distal anal canal relatively unsupported [66]. In theory, preoperative identification of such patients may define those patients likely to fare badly after conventional sphincterotomy and perhaps lead either to formal fissurectomy and advancement anoplasty rather than sphincterotomy or to more limited sphincterotomies or controlled balloon sphincter distension [67]. Prospective data is currently lacking to back up this surgical decision making, which is guided by preoperative manometry and endosonography.

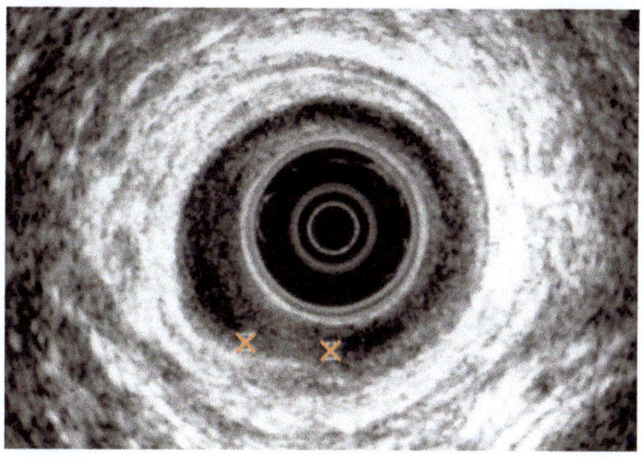

Fig. 52. Left lateral internal sphincterotomy for anal fissure (*markers*)

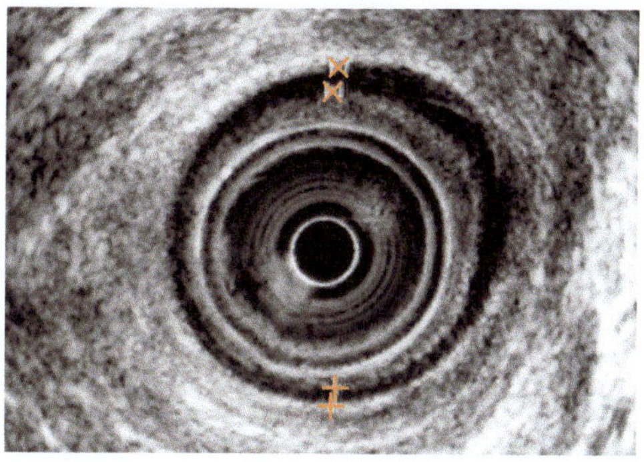

Fig. 53. Patient with a chronic anal fissure and a thin internal anal sphincter (*markers*). This patient had marked resting hypertonia on anal manometry justifying a formal internal anal sphincterotomy

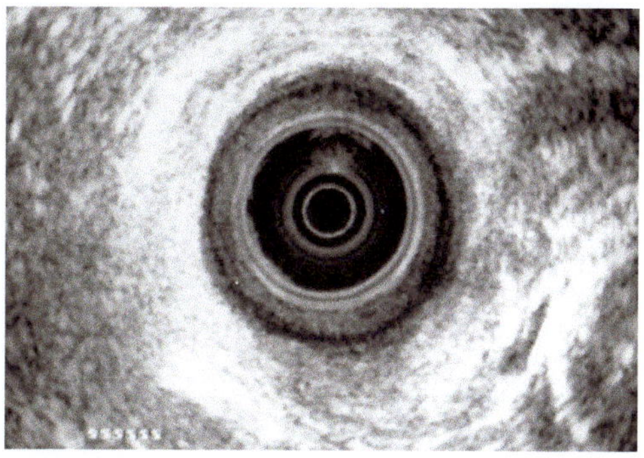

Fig. 54. Another case with internal sphincter thinner than normal with hypertone at anal manometry

Proctalgia

Proctalgia may be accompanied by many other anal lesions such as deep-seated perianal sepsis, which are readily demonstrable on endoanal ultrasonography and which require treatment in their own right. Endosonography assists the clinician in defining the organic causes for proctalgia where in patients with longstanding pain it is recognized that there is a high incidence of underlying psychological problems which present as an anal somatization disorder, frequently with a high incidence of childhood sexual abuse [68-70].

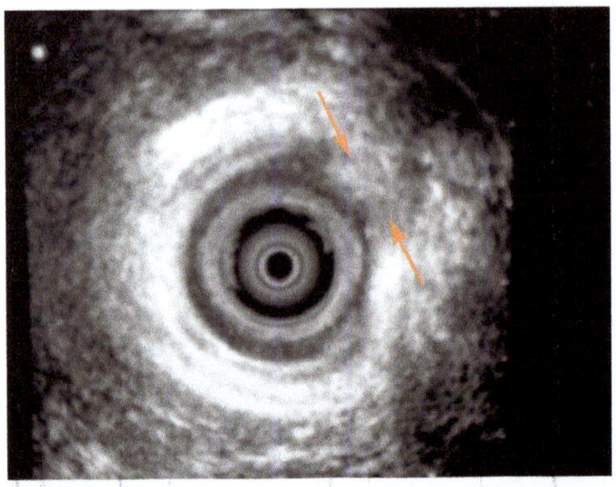

Fig. 55. Endoanal ultrasound, upper third of the anal canal. Anterior lesion of deep external sphincters (*arrows*) is evident. The internal sphincter is thin anteriorly. The patient is multiparous and has a prolonged PNTML (pudendal nerve motor latency). She also has moderate fecal incontinence (C2 Pescatori grade, score 5), with weekly loss of liquid stool

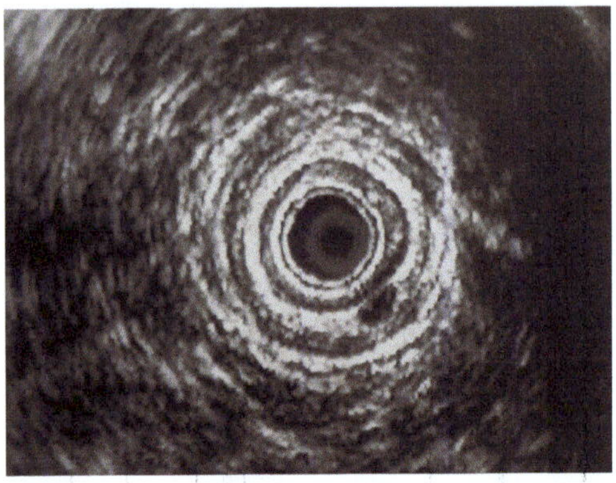

Fig. 56. A left anterolateral intersphincteric abscess in a patient with acute anal pain

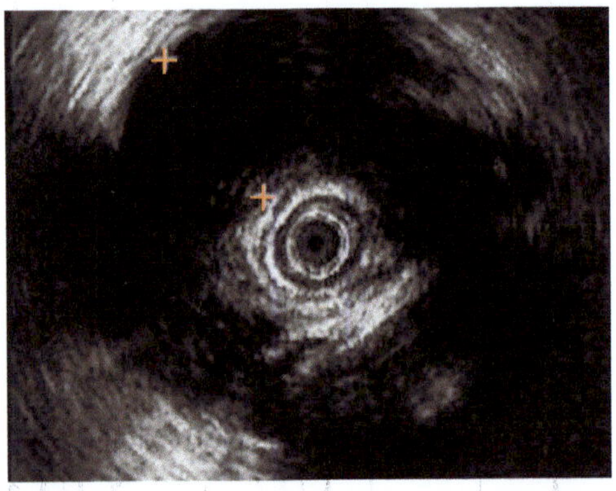

Fig. 57. A cystic ovarian carcinoma presenting with chronic anal and rectal pain (*markers*)

References

1. Beynon J, Foy DMA, Channer JL, Temple LN, Virjee J, Mortensen NJMcC (1986) The endosonic appearances of normal colon and rectum. Dis Colon Rectum 29:810-813
2. Law PJ, Bartram CI (1989) Anal endosonography: technique and normal anatomy. Gastrointest Radiol 14:349-353
3. Sultan AH, Nicholls RJ, Kamm MA, Hudson CN, Beynon J, Bartram CI (1993) Anal endosonography and correlation with in vitro and in vivo anatomy. Br J Surg 80:508-511
4. Bartram CI, Frudinger A (1997) Handbook of Anal Endosonography. Wrightson Biomedical Publishing, UK
5. Sultan AH, Kamm MA, Hudson CN, Nicholls JR, Bartram CI (1994) Endosonography of the anal sphincters: normal anatomy and comparison with manometry. Clin Radiol 49:368-374
6. Sultan AH, Loder PB, Bartram CI, Kamm MA, Hudson CN (1994) Vaginal endosonography new approach to image the undisturbed anal sphincter. Dis Colon Rectum 37:1296-1299
7. Sandridge DA, Thorp JM Jr (1995) Vaginal endosonography in the assessment of the anorectum. Obstet Gynecol 86:1007-1009
8. Alexander AR, Liu J, Menton DA, Nagle DA (1996) Fecal incontinence: transvaginal ultrasound evaluation of anatomic causes. Radiology 199:529-532
9. Frudinger A, Bartram CI, Kamm MA (1997) Transvaginal versus anal endosonography for detecting damage to the anal sphincter. Am J Roentgenol (AJR) 168:1435-1438
10. Stewart L, Wilson SR (1999) Transvaginal sonography of the anal sphincter: reliable or not? Am J Roentgenol (AJR) 173:179-185
11. Frudinger A, Zbar AP (2005) Transvaginal endosonography in the assessment of the anorectal sphincter. In: Wexner SD, Zbar AP, Pescatori M (eds) Complex Anorectal Disorders: Investigation and Management. Springer-Verlag, London, pp 258-262
12. Burnett SJ, Bartram CI (1991) Endosonographic variations in the normal internal anal sphincter. Int J Colorect Dis 6:2-4
13. Sangwan YP, Rosen L, Riether RD, Stasik JJ, Sheets JA, Khubchandani IT (1994) Is simple fistula-in-ano simple? Dis Colon Rectum 37:885-889
14. Zbar AP, deSouza NM (1999) Prospective comparison of endosonography, magnetic resonance imaging and surgical findings in anorectal fistula and abscess complicating Crohn's disease. Br J Surg 86:1093-1094
15. Abbasakoor F, Nelson M, Beynon J, Patel B, Carr ND (1998) Anal endosonography in patients with anorectal symptoms after hemorrhoidectomy. Br J Surg 85:1522-1524
16. Stoker J, Rociu, Schouten WR, Lameris JS (2002) Anovaginal and rectovaginal fistulas: endoluminal sonography versus endoluminal MR imaging. Am J Roentgenol (AJR) 178:737-741
17. Sultan AH, Kamm MA, Hudson CN, Thomas JM, Bartram CI (1993) Anal-sphincter disruption during vaginal delivery. N Engl J Med 329:1905-1911
18. Bollard RC, Gardiner A, Lindow S, Phillips RKS, Duthie GS (2002) Normal female anal sphincter: difficulties in interpretation explained. Dis Colon Rectum 45:171-175
19. Deen KI, Kumar D, Willaims JG, Oluff J, Keighley MR (1993) Anal sphincter defects: correlation between endoanal ultrasound and surgery. Ann Surg 218:201-205
20. Hill J, Hosker G, Kiff ES (2002) Pudendal nerve terminal motor latency measurements: what they do and do not tell us. Br J Surg 89:1268-1269
21. Leroi AM, Kamm MA, Weber J, Denis P, Hawley PR (1997) Internal anal sphincter repair. Int J Colorectal Dis 12:243-245
22. Gold DM, Bartram CI, Halligan S, Humphries KN, Kamm MA, Kmiot WA (1999) 3-D endoanal sonography in assessing anal canal injury. Br J Surg 86:365-370
23. Briel JW, Stoker J, Rociu E, Laméris JS, Hop WC, Schouten WR (1999) External anal sphincter atrophy on endoanal magnetic resonance imaging adversely affects continence after sphincteroplasty. Br J Surg 86:1322-1327
24. Meyer A, Hohfeld P, Actari C, Russolo A, De Grandi P (2000) Birth trauma: short and long term effects of forceps delivery compared with spontaneous delivery on various pelvic floor parameters. Br J Obstet Gynaecol 107:1360-1365

25. Donnelly V, Fynes M, Campbell D, Johnson H, O'Connell R, O'Herlihy C (1998) Obstetric events leading to anal sphincter damage. Obstet Gynecol 92:955-961
26. Samuelsson RJ, Ladifos L, Wennerholm UB, Gareberg B, Nyberg K, Hagberg H (2000) Anal sphincter tears: prospective study of obstetric risk factors. Br J Obstet Gynaecol 107:926-931
27. Faltin DL, Boulvain M, Trion O, Bretones S, Stan C, Weil A (2000) Diagnosis of anal sphincter tears by postpartum endosonography to predict fecal incontinence. Obstet Gynecol 95:643-647
28. Burnett SJ, Spence-Jones C, Speakman CT, Kamm MA, Hudson CN, Bartram CI (1991) Unsuspected sphincter damage following childbirth revealed by anal endosonography. Br J Radiol 64:225-227
29. Starck M, Bohe M, Valentin L (2003) Results of endosonographic imaging of the anal sphincter 2-7 days after primary repair of 3rd or 4th degree obstetric sphincter tears. Ultrasound Obstet Gynecol 22:609-615
30. Vaizey CJ, Kamm MA (2005) Injectable bulking agents for treating faecal incontinence. Br J Surg 92:521-527
31. Davis K, Kumar D, Poloniecki J (2003) Preliminary evaluation of an injectal sphincter bulking agent (durasphere) in the management of faecal incontinence. Aliment Pharmacol Ther 18:237-243
32. Kenefick NJ, Vaizey CJ, Malouf AJ, Norton CS, Marshall M, Kamm MA (2002) Injectable silicone biomaterial for faecal incontinenc due to internal anal sphincter dysfunction. Gut 51:225-228
33. Kumar D, Benson MJ, Bland JE (1998) Glutaraldehyde cross-linked collagen in the treatment of faecal incontinence. Br J Surg 85:978-979
34. Shafik A (1995) Perianal injection of autologous fat for treatment of sphincteric incontinence. Dis Colon Rectum 38:583-587
35. Spencer JA, Ward J, Beckingham IJ, Adams C, Ambrose NS (1996) Dynamic contrast-enhanced MR imaging of perianal fistulas. Am J Roentgenol (AJR) 167:735-741
36. Stoker J, Hussain SM, van Kempen D, Elevelt AJ, Laméris JS (1996) Endoanal coil MR imaging of anal fistulas. Am J Roentgenol (AJR) 166:360-362
37. Zbar AP, deSouza NM, Puni R, Kmiot WA (1998) Comparison of endoanal magnetic resonance imaging with surgical findings in perirectal sepsis. Br J Surg 85:111-114
38. Felt-Bersma RJ, van Baren R, Koorevaar M, Strijers RL, Cuesta MA (1995) Unsuspected sphincter defects shown by anal endosonography after anorectal surgery. A prospective study. Dis Colon Rectum 38:249-253
39. Dodi G, Pietroletti R, Milito G, Binda G, Pescatori M (2003) Bleeding, incontinence, pain and constipation after STARR transanal double stapling rectotomy for obstructed defecation. Tech Coloproctol 7:148-153
40. Abbasakoor F, Neslon M, Beynon J, Patel B, Carr ND (1998) Anal endosonography in patients with anorectal symptoms after hemorrhoidectomy. Br J Surg 85:1522-1524
41. Zbar AP, Beer-Gabel M, Chiappa AC, Aslam M (2001) Fecal incontinence after minor anorectal surgery. Dis Colon Rectum 44:1610-1623
42. Cheetham MJ, Mortensen NJ, Nystrom PO, Kamm MA, Phillips RKS (2000) Persistent pain and faecal urgency after stapled hemorrhoidectomy. Lancet 26:730-733
43. Cruiskshank SH (1991) Sacrospinous fixation-should this be performed at the time of vaginal hysterectomy? Am J Obstet Gynecol 164:1072-1076
44. Backer MH (1992) Success with sacrospinous suspension of the prolapsed vaginal vault. Surg Gynecol Obstet 175:419-420
45. McCall ML (1997) Posterior culdoplasty: surgical correction of enterocele during vaginal hysterectomy. A preliminary report. Obstet Gynecol 10:596-602
46. Lieneman A, Anthuber C, Baron A, Resier M (2000) Diagnosing enteroc`eles using dynamic magnetic resonance imaging. Dis Colon Rectum 43:205-213
47. Beer-Gabel M, Teshler M, Schechtman E, Zbar AP (2004) Dynamic transperineal ultrasound versus defecography in patients with evacuatory difficulty: a pilot study. Int J Colorectal Dis 19:60-67
48. Sitzler PJ, Kamm MA, Nicholls RJ, McKee RF (1999) Long-term clinical outcome of surgery for solitary rectal ulcer syndrome. Br J Surg 85:1246-1250

49. Kang YS, Kamm MA, Engel AF, Talbot IC (1996) Pathology of the rectal wall in solitary rectal ulcer syndrome and complete rectal prolapse. Gut 38:587-590
50. Pescatori M, Quondamcarlo C (1999) A new grading of rectal internal mucosal prolapse and its correlation with diagnosis and treatment. Int J Colorectal Dis 14:245-249
51. Pescatori M, Favetta U, Dedola S, Orsini S (1997) Transanal stapled excision of rectal mucosal prolapse. Tech Coloproctol 1:96-98
52. Pescatori M, Boffi F, Russo A, Zbar AP (2005) Complications and recurrence after excision of rectal internal mucosal prolapse for obstructed defecation. Int J Colorectal Dis 7:107-108
53. Jones PN, Lubowski DZ, Swash M, Henry MM (1987) Is paradoxical contraction of the puborectalis muscle of functional importance? Dis Colon Rectum 30:667-670
54. Fleshman JW, Dreznik Z, Cohen E, Fry RD, Kodner IJ (1992) Balloon expulsion test facilitates diagnosis of pelvic floor outlet obstruction due to nonrelaxing puborectalis muscle. Dis Colon Rectum 35:1019-1025
55. Ger GC, Wexner SD, Jorge JM, Salanga VD (1993) Anorectal manometry in the diagnosis of paradoxical puborectalis syndrome. Dis Colon Rectum 36:816-825
56. Jorge JM, Wexner SD, Ger GC, Salanga VD, Nogueras JJ, Jagelman DG (1993) Cinedefecography and electromyography in the diagnosis of nonrelaxing puborectalis syndrome. Dis Colon Rectum 36:668-676
57. Nehra V, Bruce BK, Rath-Harvey DM, Pemberton JH, Camilleri M (2000) Psychological disorders in patients with evacuation disorders and constipation in a tertiary practice. Am J Gastroenterol 95:1755-1758
58. Kraft R (1962) Duplication anomalies of the rectum. Ann Surg 155:230-232
59. Alavanja G, Kaderabek DJ, Habegger ED (1995) Rectal duplication in an adult. Am Surg 61:997-1000
60. Flint R, Strang J, Bissett I, Clark M, Neill M, Parry B (2004) Rectal duplication cyst presenting as perianal sepsis: report of two cases and review of the literature. Dis Colon Rectum 47:2208-2210
61. deSouza NM, Ward HC, Willaims AD, Battin M, Harris DNF, McIver DK (1999) Transanal MR imaging after repair of anorectal anomalies in children: appearances in pullthrough vs. Posterior sagittal reconstructions. Am J Roentgenol (AJR) 173:723-728
62. Sultan AH, Kamm MA, Nicholls RJ, Bartram CI (1994) Prospective study of the extent of lateral anal sphincterotomy division during lateral sphincterotomy. Dis Colon Rectum 37:1031-1033
63. Nyam DC, Pemberton JH (1999) Long-term results of lateral internal sphincterotomy for chronic anal fissure with particular reference to incidence of fecal incontinence. Dis Colon Rectum 42:1306-1320
64. Zbar AP, Aslam M, Allgar V (2000) Faecal incontinence after internal sphincterotomy for anal fissure. Tech Coloproctol 4:25-28
65. Zbar AP, Kmiot WA, Aslam M, Williams A, Hider A, Audisio RA, Chiappa AC, deSouza NM (1999) Use of vector volume manometry and endoanal magnetic resonance imaging in the adult female for assessment of anal sphincter dysfunction. Dis Colon Rectum 42:1411-1418
66. Pescatori M, Maria G, Anastasio G (1991) "Spasm related" internal sphincterotomy in treatment of anal fissure. A randomized prospective study. Coloproctology 1:20-22
67. Renzi A, Brusciano L, Pescatori M et al (2005) Pneumatic balloon dilatation for chronic anal fissure. A prospective clinical endosonographic and manometric trial. Dis Colon Rectum 47:1846-1851
68. Leroi AM, Bernier C, Watier A (1995) Prevalence of sexual abuse among patients with functional disorders of the lower gastrointestinal tract. Int J Colorectal Dis 10:200-206
69. Renzi C, Pescatori M (2000) Psychologic aspects in proctalgia. Dis Colon Rectum 43:535-539
70. Russo A, Pescatori M (2005) Psychological assessment of patients with proctological disorders. In: Wexner SD, Zbar AP, Pescatori M (eds). Complex Anorectal Disorders: Investigation and Management. Springer-Verlag, London, pp 747-760

3 Three-Dimensional Endoanal Ultrasound in Benign Proctological Practice

Clive I. Bartram, Mario Pescatori

Introduction

Magnetic resonance (MR) imaging of the anal sphincters has shown the advantages inherent in multiplanar imaging, notable determining the length of the sphincters, relating the cranial extent of sepsis to the levators [1] and determining the adequacy of external anal sphincteroplasty [2].

Design variations in conventional endoanal axial sonography have permitted the acquisition of multiple images with sequential short-step probe withdrawal and a video capture card to obtain a coherent dataset, with proprietary 3-dimensional software to analyse the dataset [3]. Such an approach has confirmed the inherent gender differences in the normal anal canal [4], has been used in patients with fecal incontinence, where there is a correlation between the angle and the coronal length of the external anal sphincter defect [5] as well as in complicated perirectal sepsis [6].

Using a recently developed commercial system that is fully automated for data acquisition and interpretation, rapid 3D image evaluation has been possible and has shown that hydrogen peroxide enhancement of fistulous tracks has no advantage in the detection of secondary tracks or ancillary abscesses, and with 3D where is better delineation of the presence and site of the internal opening [7].

Three dimensional endoanal reconstructed ultrasonography still has the same inherent limitations of 2-D endosonography in regard to resolution and tissue contrast in the axial plane, and in the "Z" axis the resolution will be inferior unless the voxel size is isometric. Penetration depends on transducer frequency.

The technical conduct of 3-D endoanal sonography is different to that of a 2-D examination, as interpretation and diagnosis does not have to be made in real-time. Even if a large number of images are recorded in 2D, these are seldom sufficient for accurate review, whereas with a 3D examination once a dataset of adequate quality has been acquired, it may be reviewed at leisure and going backwards and forwards through the dataset gives as much information as when the examination was being first performed. Acquisition may therefore be separated from diagnosis and could easily be performed by technicians. The latest endoprobe design, the type 2050 transducer, from B-K Medical (B-K Medical, Herlev, Denmark) is designed specifically for 3D endosonography. There is no external moving part and two back-to-back multifrequency 6-16 MHz crystals are mechanically rotated and pulled back within the probe housing, so that the probe does not actually move within the anal canal, minimising any artefact. The speed of rotation may be varied, but scans are performed usually at 9 frames per sec giving a linear transducer movement of 2.25 mm/sec and a total scan time of 15-20 sec to obtain complete coverage of the anal canal. The 3D software is fully integrated into the system and reformats the dataset rapidly to allow almost immediate confirmation of the technical adequacy of the examination. The dataset may be reviewed in any plane. The pixel size is 0.13 mm in the X and Y axis, but 0.25 mm in the Z axis, so that resolution is reduced slightly in the coronal and sagittal planes. Measurements are possible in any plane, and the volume may be rendered to improve conspicuity of difficult areas.

Normal Anatomy

The normal anatomy on 3D has been described [3] and the layers of the anal sphincter complex defined sonographically and proven by comparison to MRI. Multiplanar imaging is particularly helpful to measure the length of the internal sphincter, to distinguish the puboanalis, its fusion with the longitudinal muscle of the rectum and to trace the extent of the conjoined muscle in the longitudinal layer, as well as demonstrating the fusion of the transverse perineii into anterior aspect of the external sphincter in women. This part of the external sphincter is seen best in the coronal plane, and is a useful view to asses its integrity.

Attempts have been made utilizing 3-D endosonography to equate the morphological representation of the sphincteric muscles with their physiological contribution to basal and squeeze pressure [4]. However, the finding that a high pressure zone extends at rest below the internal anal sphincter termination is at variance with anal vector-volumetry where there was no difference in resting HPZ length between continent and incontinent cohorts of patients after equivalent length lateral internal sphincterotomy [8]. There may be disparity between how the muscle group limits are described [9] and the manometric zones, and the differences between sphincter lengths in the sexes as shown also by MR imaging [10, 11] adds to the complexity of attempts to correlate structure with function. Nevertheless, the 3-D data that the puborectalis muscle occupies a significantly larger proportion of the anal canal in women without any fundamental gender differences in internal anal sphincter length may be important where internal anal sphincterotomy is to be performed (resistant chronic anal fissure), or where both internal and external anal sphincter muscle is to be deliberately sacrificed (trans-sphincteric fistulotomy). An improved understanding of the normal gender differences in the anal canal utilizing 3-D endoanal sonography and the functional relevance of these will assist in the interpretation of pathological and postoperative states.

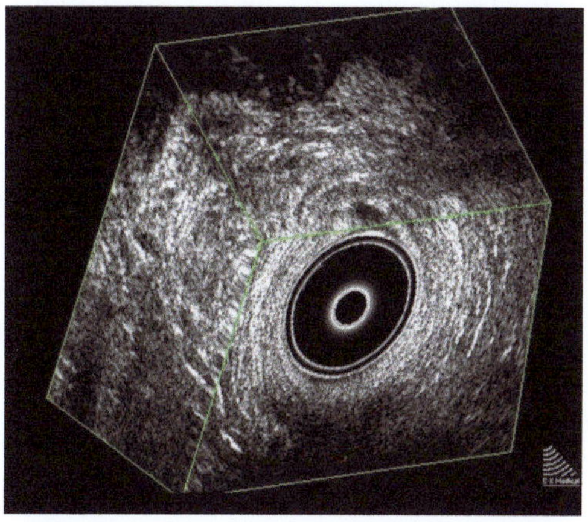

Fig. 58a. The normal appearance of the external anal sphincter complex using 3-D endosonography does not provide the typical subdivisions (deep, superficial and subcutaneous) which are seen in coronal views with endoanal MR imaging

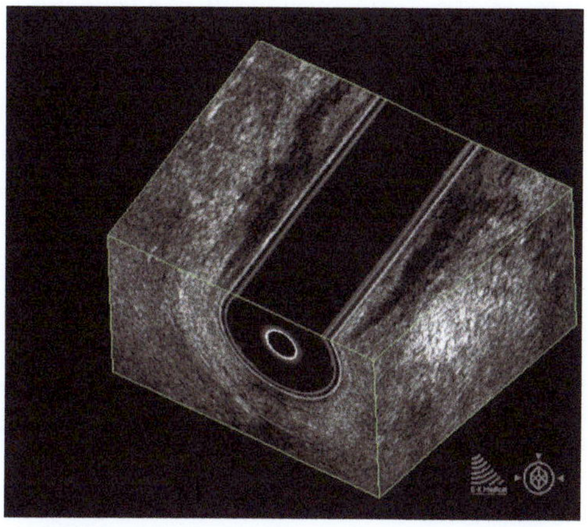

Fig. 58b. Coronal reconstruction over the entire length of the normal female anal canal. This shows the termination of the internal anal sphincter and the constitutive nature of the external/internal anal sphincter overlap in the distal anal canal. The external anal sphincter has been shown to be longer in males as part of an overall-longer anal canal with a mean internal anal sphincter: total anal canal ratio that is equivalent between the sexes

Figures provided by courtesy of Dr. A. Frudinger, Graz, Austria and reproduced with permission from [12]

Fecal Incontinence

Three-dimensional anal endosonography may provide some important information regarding the layout of the sphincters (even when damaged) that may assist the surgical planning of sphincteroplasty [13] based on the comparability of 3-D reconstructed images to those obtained in the coronal plane with endoanal MR imaging [14, 15]. Poor functional outcome after external anal sphincteroplasty may arise from a failure to oppose sufficient length of the sphincter in the repair (or the incorporation of an attendant levatorplasty). Another consideration during pelvic floor repair is that the overzealous mobilization of the external anal sphincter may result in devascularization and denervation of the external sphincter [16]. Here, Gold and colleagues have shown a correlation between the proximal extent of an external anal sphincter defect and its angle of separation [2] which tells the surgeon that wider defects are likely to be longer, governing the conduct of the initial sphincteroplasty. This would also correlate with the finding that most failed external anal sphincteroplasties show persistent defects on conventional endosonography [17]. The clinical impact of 3-D technology on repeat sphincteroplasty has yet to be determined [18, 19]. The role of external anal sphincter atrophy on repair, as demonstrated endoanal MR imaging [20] is also a cause of poor outcome to sphincteroplasty. Passive incontinence from either intentional internal anal sphincter division, injudicious injury to the sphincter by manual dilatation or the extended use of an endoanal retractor [21, 22] may be assessed accurately by 3-D endosonography, with not only the radial extent of sphincter damage, but also its linear extent and percentage involvement of the sphincter calculated. Lateral internal anal sphincterotomy is particularly a problem in women, where its extent may be greater than intended [23].

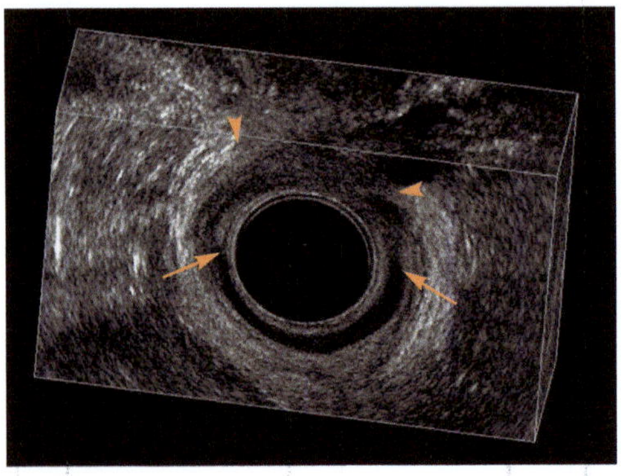

Fig. 59. Obstetric trauma with a well defined external anal sphincter tear between the 12 o'clock and 2 o'clock positions (*arrowheads*) and in the internal anal sphincter between the 9 o'clock and 3 o'clock positions (*arrows*) seen both axially and coronally in the 3-D image. Note the asymmetry of the anterior ring of the external sphincter due to the left sided tear, which is best appreciated in the coronal component of the image afforded by the 3-D reconstructed view

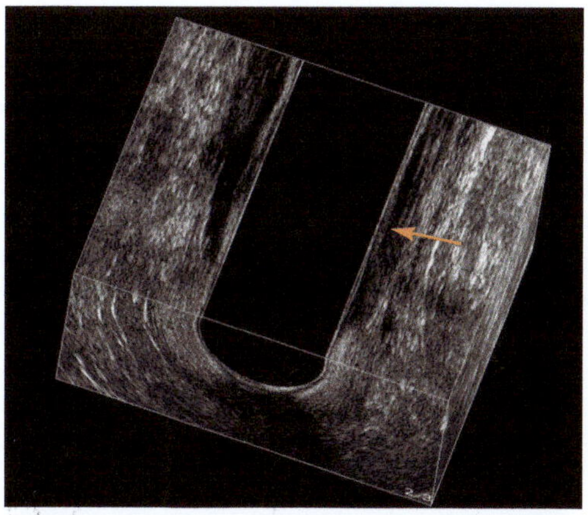

Fig. 60. The appearance after lateral internal anal sphincterotomy seen in coronal section. The length of the internal anal sphincter and the percentage of sphincter divided can be estimated (in this case 31% of the total internal anal sphincter length). Low reflective scarring is seen in the plane of the internal anal sphincter below its point of division when compared to the contralateral side (*arrow*)

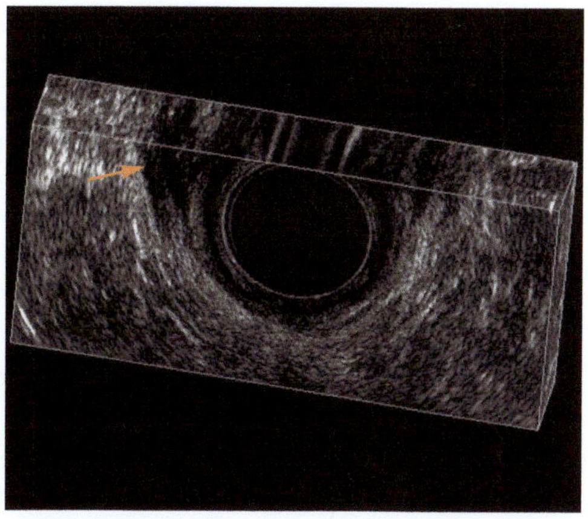

Fig. 61. Example of extensive obstetric sphincter trauma shows a tear in the right puboanalis muscle extending into the longitudinal muscle layer coronally (*arrow*)

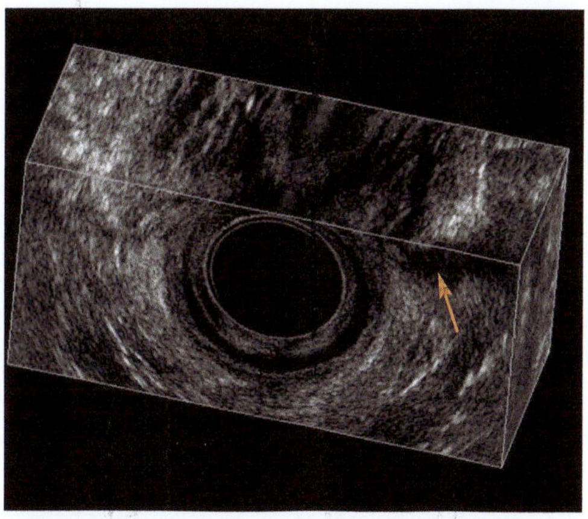

Fig. 62. The figure represents a tear in the left transverse perinei as appreciated axially (*arrow*) along with a concomitant tear in the external anal sphincter

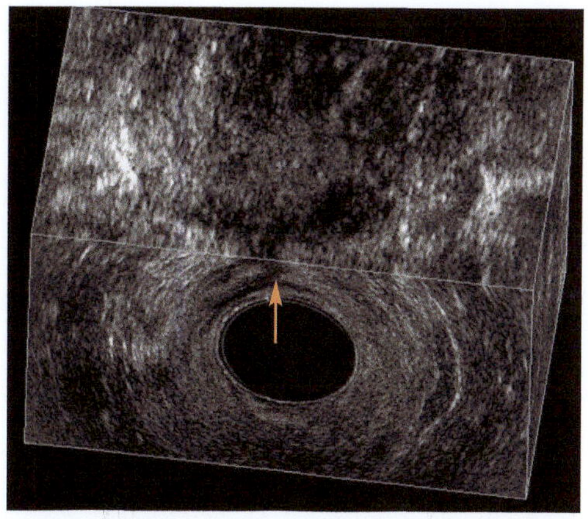

Fig. 63. This figure shows how this anterior external anal sphincter defect is best appreciated on the coronal 3-D image (*arrow*)

Anal Fistula and Abscess

Two-dimensional endoanal sonography has proven value in its surgical correlation for complex perianal sepsis [24] and for rectovaginal fistula [25], despite some limitations in the demonstration of supralevator and extrasphincteric disease as well as in the separation of active recrudescent sepsis from burnt-out disease. Three-dimensional reconstructed images are more readily able to trace the extent and direction of tracks and collections within the infra-levator and supra-levator (if a water filled balloon is used to obtain acoustic contact within the distal rectum) compartments, and provide a visual representation of the fistula track in an anatomical plane that is more akin to the surgical approach than those images traditionally provided by an axial view. There is some evidence to suggest that 3-D endosonography is better than conventional endosonography in demonstrating the site of the internal opening [7]. The prospective predictive role of 3-D endosonography in anal fistula management, and in the prevention of fistula recurrence through its impact on surgical treatment, remains to be defined.

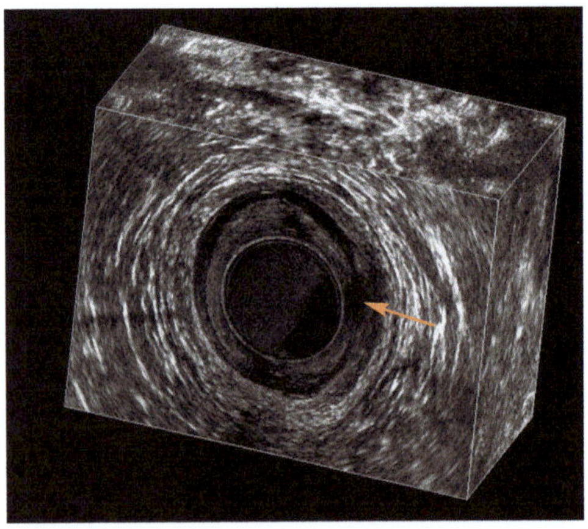

Fig. 64a. Axial view of a low anal fistula showing the internal opening at the 3 o'clock position (*arrow*)

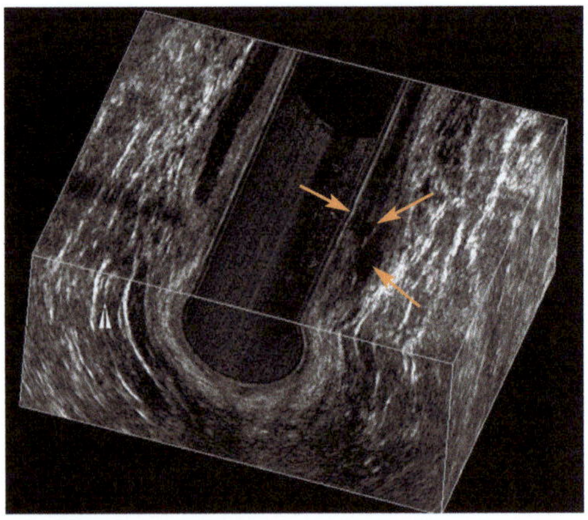

Fig. 64b. A reconstructed coronal view where the pathway of the fistula can be readily traced through the internal anal sphincter to the point of its internal opening (*arrows*). The internal anal sphincter in this case is not seen as a typically low reflective structure immediately adjacent to the fistula since it has become more reflective as a result of inflammatory change

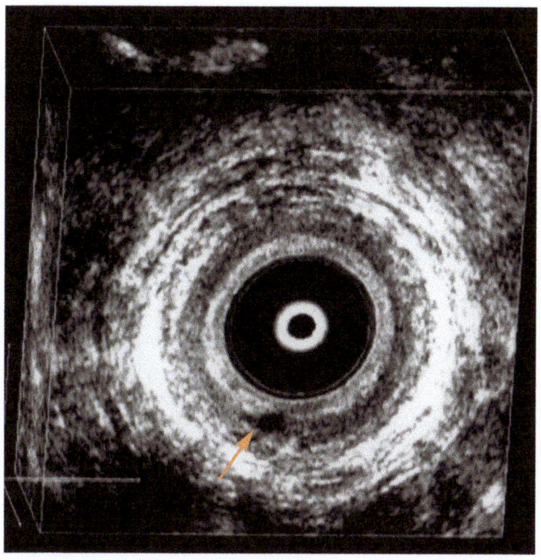

Fig. 65a. 3-D endoanal ultrasound of middle third anal canal (coronal view): anal fistula passing through the inter- anal sphincter (*arrows*)

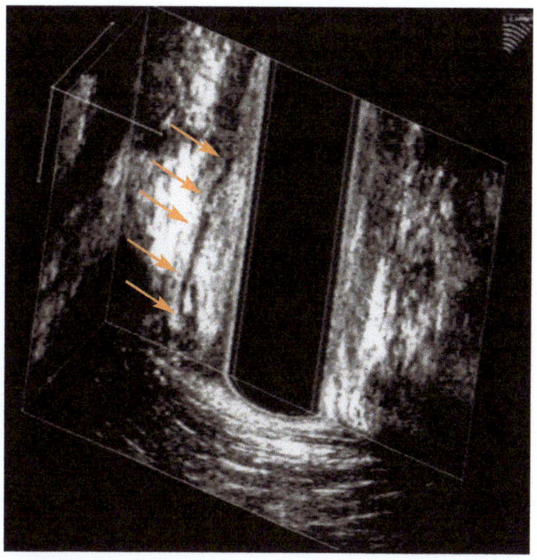

Fig. 65b. 3-D endoanal ultrasound of same fistula (longitudinal view): trans-sphincteric tract is indicated by arrows

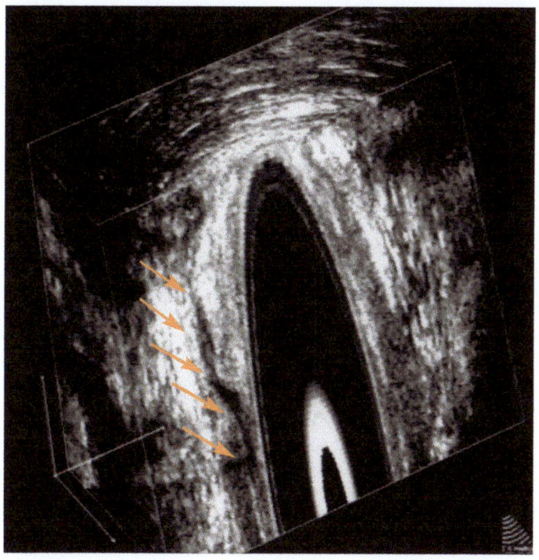

Fig. 65c. 3-D endoanal ultrasound of same fistula (oblique view): trans-sphincteric tract is indicated by *arrows* (Courtesy of C. Ratto)

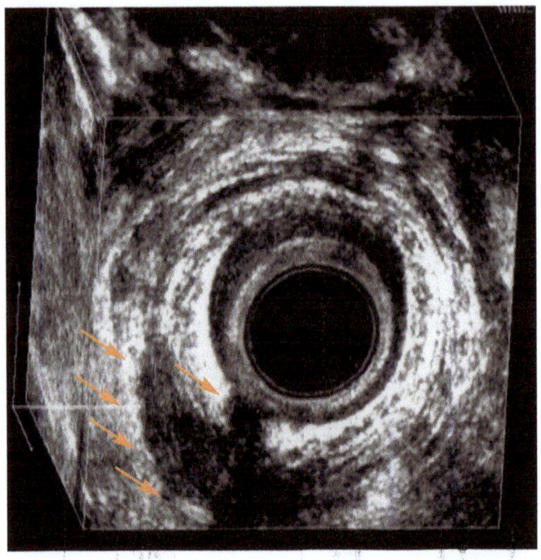

Fig. 66a. 3-D endoanal ultrasound of anal abscess with trans-sphincteric primary tract, indicated by *arrows*: coronal view

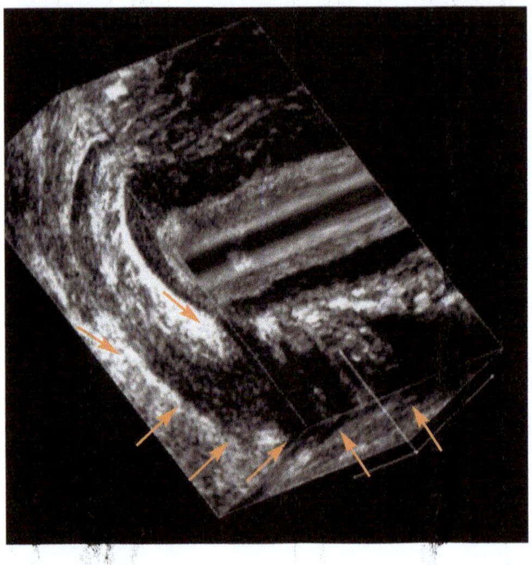

Fig. 66b. Longitudinal view of the same case (Courtesy of C. Ratto)

Constipation and Proctalgia

Three-dimensional endosonography has a role in the assessment of a range of benign proctological disorders, and a developing one in proctalgia where patients may have unrecognized sepsis or rare conditions such as hereditary internal anal sphincter myopathy. In this condition the internal anal sphincter is grossly thickened (>6 mm) and from excision biopsy at myotomy will be found to contain PAS-positive cytoplasmic inclusions and ultrastructural changes on electron microscopy resembling other isolated polyglucosan storage myopathies, including adult polyglucosan disease and Lafora's disease [26-29].

The internal anal sphincter increases in thickness with advancing age [30]. In adults it is normally 2-3 mm. Thickening in the range 3-6 mm throughout the sphincter, as shown on 3D multiplanar views, is uncommon is simple constipation, and has a high predictive value for rectal prolapse or intra-anal intussusception [31]. With advanced prolapse the internal sphincter may be thickened but fragmented by distension from the prolapse.

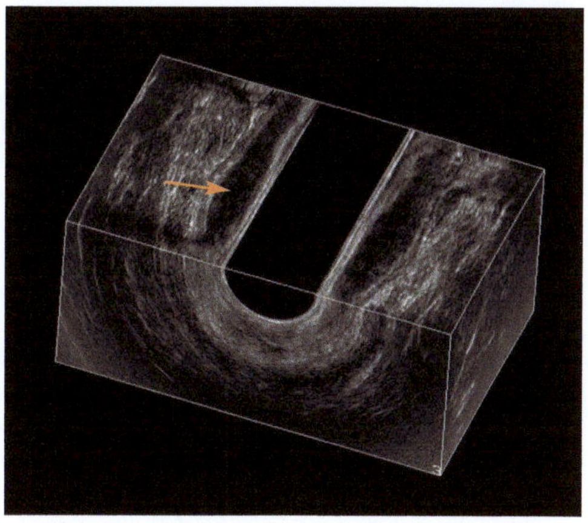

Fig. 67. An abnormally thick internal anal sphincter (5 mm) is shown in this coronal 3-D reconstruction (*arrow*). The patient was a 43 year-old woman who presented with obstructed defecation and proctalgia

References

1. Barker PG, Lunniss PJ, Armstrong P, Reznek RH, Cottam K, Phillips RKS (1994) Magnetic resonance imaging of fistula-in-ano: technique, interpretation and accuracy. Clin Radiol 49:7-13
2. Gold DM, Bartram CI, Halligan S, Humphries KN, Kamm MA, Kmiot WA (1999) 3-D endoanal sonography in assessing anal canal injury. Br J Surg 86:365-370
3. Williams AB, Bartram CI, Halligan S, Marshall MM, Nicholls RJ, Kmiot WA (2001) Multiplanar anal endosonography - normal canal anatomy. Colorectal Dis 3:169-174
4. Williams AB, Cheetham MJ, Bartram CI, Halligan S, Kam MA, Nicholls RJ, Kmiot WA (2000) Gender differences in the longitudinal pressure profile of the anal canal related to anatomical structure as demonstrated on three-dimensional anal endosonography. Br J Surg 87:1674-1679
5. Williams AB, Bartram I, Halligan S, Marshall MM, Spencer JA, Nicholls RJ, Kmiot WA (2002) Alteraton of anal sphincter morphology following vaginal delivery revealed by multiplanar anal endosonography. BJOG 109:942-946
6. West RI, Zimmerman DDE, Dwarkasing S, Hop WCJ, Hussain SM, Schouten WR, Kuipers EJ, Felt-Bersma RJ (2003) Prospective comparison of hydrogen peroxide-enhanced 3-D endoanal ultrasonography and endoanal MR imaging of perianal fistulas. Dis Colon Rectum 46:1407-1415
7. Buchanan GN, Bartram CI, Williams AB, Halligan S, Cohen CR (2005) Value of hydrogen peroxide enhancement of three-dimensional endoanal ultrasound in fistula-in-ano. Dis Colon Rectum 48:141-147
8. Zbar AP, Beer-Gabel M, Chiappa AC, Aslam M (2001) Fecal incontinence after minor anoectal surgery. Dis Colon Rectum 44:1610-1623
9. Fucini C, Elbetti C, Messerini L (1999) Anatomic plane of separation between external anal sphincter and puborectalis muscle: clinical implications. Dis Colon Rectum 42:374-379
10. deSouza NM, Puni R, Zbar A, Gilderdale DJ, Couuts GA, Krausz T (1996) MR imaging of the anal sphincter in multiparous women using an endoanal coil: correlation with in vitro anatomy and appearances in fecal incontinence. Am J Roentgenol (AJR) 167:1465-1471
11. Zbar AP, Kmiot WA, Aslam M, Williams A, Hider A, Audisio RA, Chiappa AC, deSouza NM (1999) Use of vector volume manometry and endoanal magnetic resonance imaging in the adult female for assessment of anal sphincter dysfunction. Dis Colon Rectum 42:1411-1418
12. Wexner SD, Zbar AP, Pescatori M (2005) Complex anorectal disorders: investigation and management. Springer-Verlag, London, pp 265-266
13. Sultan AH, Kamm MA, Hudson CN, Nicholls RJ, Bartram CI (1994) Endosonography of the anal sphincters: normal anatomy and comparison with manometry. Clin Radiol 49:368-374
14. Hussain SM, Stoker J, Zwamborn AW, Den Hollander JC, Kuiper JW, Entius CA, Lameris JS (1996) Endoanal MRI of the anal sphincter complex: correlation with cross-sectional anatomy and histology. J Anat 189:677-682
15. West RL, Felt-Bersma RJ, Hansen BE, Schouten WR, Kuipers EJ (2005) Volume measurements of the anal sphincter complex in healthy controls and fecal-incontinent patients with a three-dimensional reconstruction of endoanal ultrasonography images. Dis Colon Rectum 48:540-548
16. Halverson AL, Hull TL (2002) Long-term outcome of overlapping anal sphincter repair. Dis Colon Rectum 45:345-348
17. Engel AF, Kamm MA, Sultan AH, Bartram CI, Nicholls RJ (1994) Anterior anal sphincter repair in patients with obstetric trauma. Br J Surg 81:1231-1234
18. Pinedo G, Vaizey CJ, Nicholls RJ, Roach R, Halligan S, Kamm MA (1999) Results of repeat anal sphincter repair. Br J Surg 86:66-69
19. Giordano P, Remzi A, Efron J, Gervaz P, Weiss EG, Nogueras JJ, Wexner SD (2002) Previous sphincter repair does not affect the outcome of repeat repair. Dis Colon Rectum 45:635-640
20. Briel JW, Stoker J, Rociu E, Laméris JS, Hop WC, Schouten WR (1999) External anal sphincter atrophy on endoanal magnetic resonance imaging adversely affects continence after sphincteroplasty. Br J Surg 86:1322-1327

21. van Tets WF, Kuijpers JF, Tran K, Mollen R, van Goor H (1997) Influence of Parks' anal retractor on anal sphincter pressures. Dis Colon Rectum 40:1042-1045
22. Zimmerman DD, Gosselink MP, Hop WC, Darby M, Briel JW, SchoutenWR (2003) Impact of two different tyoes of anal retractor on fecal continence after fistula repair: a prospective, randomized, clinical trial. Dis Colon Rectum 46:1674-1679
23. Sultan AH, Kamm MA, Nicholls RJ, Bartram CI (1994) Prospective study of the extent of lateral anal sphincterotomy division during lateral sphincterotomy. Dis Colon Rectum 37:1031-1033
24. Kruskal JB, Kane RA, Morrin MM (2001) Peroxide-enhanced anal endosonography: technique, image interpretation and clinical application. Radiographics 21:S173-S189
25. Lawrence FY, Birnbaum EH, Read TE, Kodner IJ, Fleshman JW (1999) Use of endoanal ultrasound in patients with rectovaginal fistulas. Dis Colon Rectum 42:1057-1064
26. Suzuki K, David E, Kutscman B (1971) Presenile dementia with 'Lafora-like' intraneuronal inclusions. Arch Neurol 25:69-80
27. Kamm MA, Hoyle CH, Burleigh DE, Law PJ, Swash M, Martin JE, Nicholls RJ, Northover JM (1991) Hereditary internal anal sphincter myopathy causing proctalgia fugax and constipation. A newly defined condition. Gastroenterology 100:805-810
28. Guy RJ, Kamm MA, Martin JE (1997) Internal anal sphincter myopathy causing proctalgia fugax and constipation: further clinical and radiological characterizaion in a patient. Eur J Gastroenterol Hepatol 9:221-224
29. de la Portilla F, Borrero JJ, Rafel E (2005) Hereditary vacuolar internal anal sphincter myopathy causing proctalgia fugax and constipation: a new case contribution. Eur J Gastroenterol Hepatol 17:359-361
30. Burnett SJ, Bartram CI (1991) Endosonographic variations in the normal internal anal sphincter. Int J Colorectal Dis 6:2-4
31. Halligan S, Malouf A, Bartram CI, Marshall M, Hallings N, Kamm MA (2001) Predictive value of impaired evacuation at proctography in diagnosis anismus. Am J Roentgenal 177:633-636

4 Static and Dynamic Transperineal Sonography in Benign Proctology

Andrew P. Zbar

Introduction

Transperineal sonography has only recently been introduced into proctological practice although it had been reported many years ago along with transintroital sonography for clinical use in urology in the assessment of bladder base descent and cystocele diagnosis in patients with urinary stress incontinence [1, 2]. The principle is simple, utilizing standard ultrasound probes for determination of the disposition of the perineal and pelvic floor soft tissues of the posterior, middle and anterior compartments by delineation of the basic bony and soft-tissue landmarks including the pubic symphisis, the urethrovesical junction, the vaginal vault, the puborectalis sling and levator floor and the anal angle. Static transperineal sonography places the probe of a basic ultrasound (either 7.5 or 10 MHz) against the perineal body in front of the anus in transverse disposition to outline the axial anal structures including the anal mucosa and submucosa and the internal and external anal sphincters and providing images which are comparable with those obtained using an endoluminal probe [3, 4]. The delineated layers of the sphincters naturally have the same echogenic characteristics as those obtained with endoanal ultrasonography with relatively poor delineation of the perineal body. The anal mucosa and submucosa are more demonstrable and Duplex sonography defines blood flow in patients with hemorrhoids and rectal mucosal prolapse, although there is as yet no specific classification system which has correlated with clinical or endoscopic grades.

Rotation of the probe through 180 degrees defines a sagittal view of the anal canal and anorectal junction showing the hypoechoic internal anal sphincter and the hyperechoic puborectalis in profile [5]. The former appears as a double dark strip on either side of the anal canal and the latter as a bright cone behind the air-filled rectum as the anal canal shifts direction. This shift in direction permits the calculation of anorectal junction movement during forcible straining or simulated evacuation and the measurement of the anorectal angle during these provocative maneuvers; both of which have been shown to correlate closely with these parameters as measured during conventional defecography [6]. The instillation of small volumes (< 50 mL) of acoustic contrast gel into both the rectum and the vagina permits better definition of these structures, allowing a dynamic representaion of the pelvic structures during straining and permitting adequate diagnosis of rectoceles, rectoanal intussusception and mucosal (or full-thickness) rectal prolapse in patients who present with evacuatory difficulty. This technique is proving invaluable as dynamic transperineal ultrasound in such patients although it remains to compare its diagnostic sensitivity of single and multiple pelvic floor pathologies with dynamic magnetic resonance (MR) imaging. Initial comparisons with standard defecography has shown good initial clinical correlation, where the use of saline or water soluble Gastrografin (Schering, UK) oral loading has been able to demonstrate coincident enteroceles [6]. The diagnosis of an enterocele in patients with rectocele as a predominant clinical finding alters the coloproctologic surgical approach and has been demonstrated as a more common finding in patients post-hysterectomy where initial culdosuspension of the vaginal vault (sacrocolpopexy) has not been performed [7, 8]. Although the relationship and pathophysiology of post-hysterectomy constipation and defecation difficulty is complex and at present poorly understood, there is an association between subsequent vaginal vault prolapse, enterocele and rectocele because of failure to obliterate the peritoneal cul-de-sac of the pouch of Douglas and to suspend the vaginal apex [9]. The presence of these concomitant disorders in rectocele patients undergoing surgery has been shown to adversely affect functional outcome if they are not surgically addressed as well as to diminish the reported efficiency after surgery of satisfactory rectal evacuation and the need for assisted defecation by perineal or vaginal pressure and manipulation [10, 11].

There is currently much prospective work that needs to be performed comparing dynamic transperineal sonography with other standard modalities in a range of pelvic floor disorders including uterovaginal prolapse, rectal prolapse and reported evacuatory 'block.' At the present time, the indications for transperineal sonography are controversial and there is a substantial learning curve in its interpretation. Transperineal sonography should be thought of as complementary to other modalities in a range of diseases. In perirectal sepsis it has an added advantage over endoanal sonography in the delineation of laterally disposed extrasphincteric fistulae which exceed the focal distance of the probe as well as in defining the upward translevator extensions of abscesses where endoluminal probes are unable to adequately couple above the puborectalis muscle [12, 13]. Such an approach may also separate perineal sepsis from perianal infection and in the definition of ano- and rectovaginal fistula extensions. In fecal incontinence, early assessment of the axial and coronal adequacy of overlapping sphincteroplasty may be performed without endoanal distraction for both intraoperative and early postoperative assessment. In specialist circumstances transperineal sonography may be the definitive modality for use including in the assessment of congenital anorectal anomalies [14] or where there is anal canal distortion which prevents the deployment of an endorectal probe.

Normal Anatomy

Figure 68 shows a typical axial view obtained using the transperineal probe. The principal point of reference is the hypoechoic ring of the internal anal sphincter and the anterior external anal sphincter usually looks fairly compressed. Figure 69 shows a sagittal transperineal ultrasound and again the landmark is the parallel hypoechoic line in profile of the internal anal sphincter.

At the right level, the puborectalis muscle is seen as a bright solid elliptical structure en face. The rectum can be filled with contrast (as can the vagina) to highlight the rectogenital septum or the rectum can be identified as an air-filled viscus. The bladder and the urethrovesical junction are readily seen anteriorly, as is the brilliantly echogenic pubis.

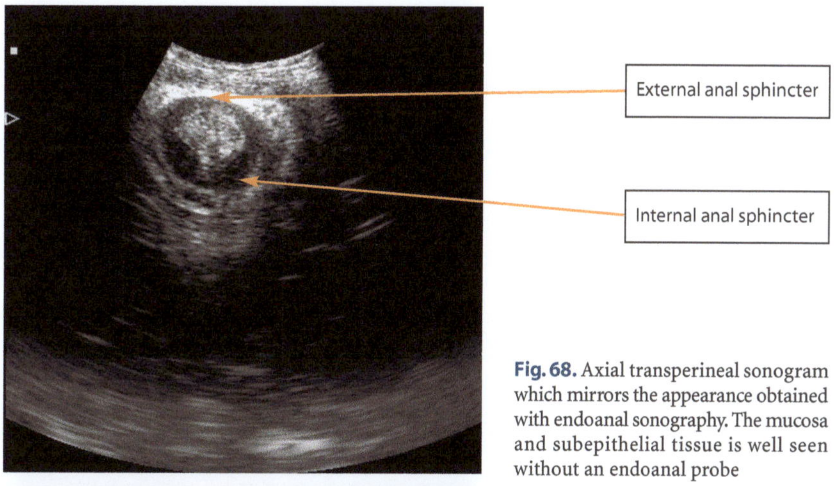

Fig. 68. Axial transperineal sonogram which mirrors the appearance obtained with endoanal sonography. The mucosa and subepithelial tissue is well seen without an endoanal probe

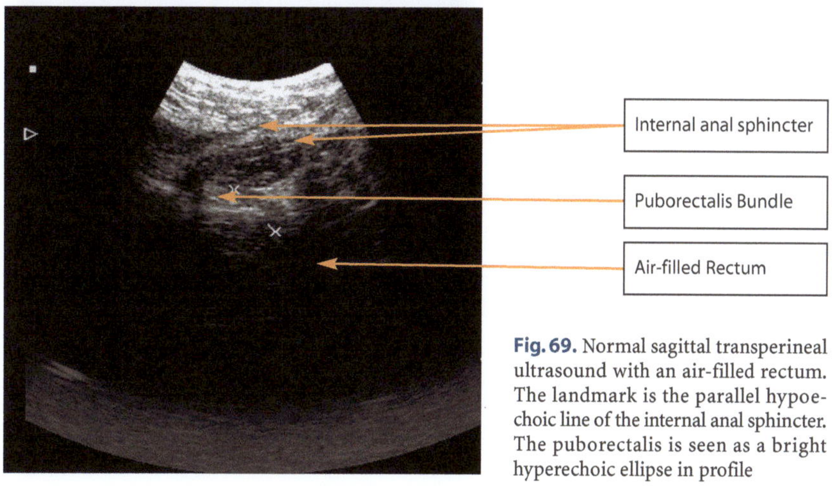

Fig. 69. Normal sagittal transperineal ultrasound with an air-filled rectum. The landmark is the parallel hypoechoic line of the internal anal sphincter. The puborectalis is seen as a bright hyperechoic ellipse in profile

Fecal Incontinence

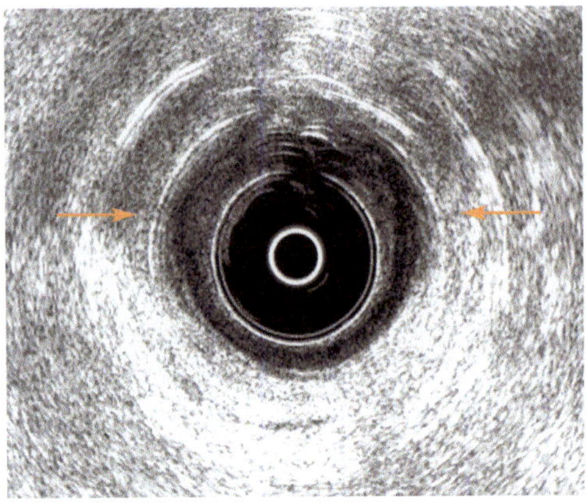

Fig. 70a. A 43 year-old woman presented 10 years after a forceps-assisted vaginal delivery with fecal incontinence. Clinical examination suggested an anterior external anal sphincter defect confirmed on endoanal ultrasound.The *arrows* show the extent of the anterior defect on sonogram.

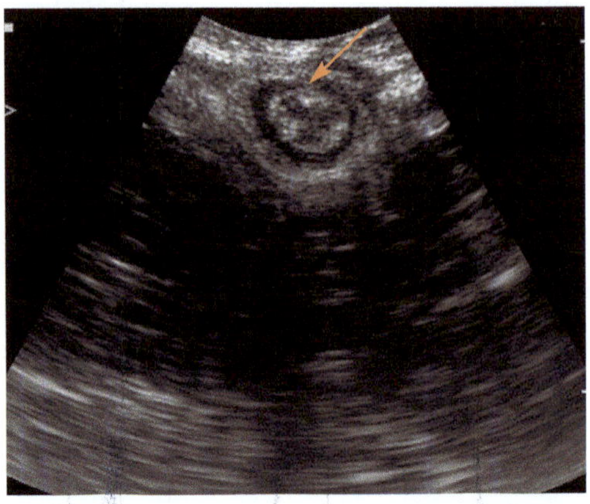

Fig. 70b. Transperineal ultrasound of the same patient. The hypoechoic circle is the internal anal sphincter, surrounded by the hyperechoic circle of the external anal sphincter seen to be deficient anteriorly (*arrow*)

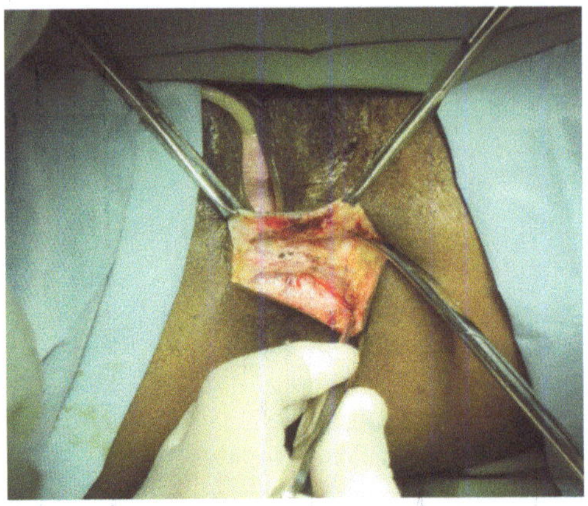

Fig. 70c. The intraoperative repair of this patient which was performed with an attendant anterior levatorplasty. The atrophic anterior external anal sphincter is exposed through a transperineal incision

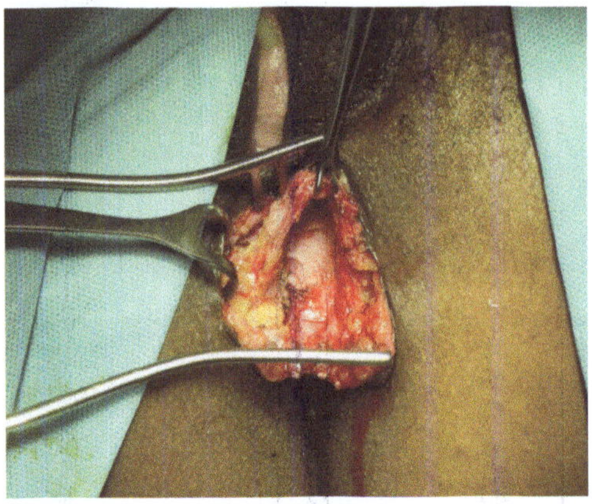

Fig. 70d. The external anal sphincter is lifted in a Babcock forcep for division and sphincteroplasty

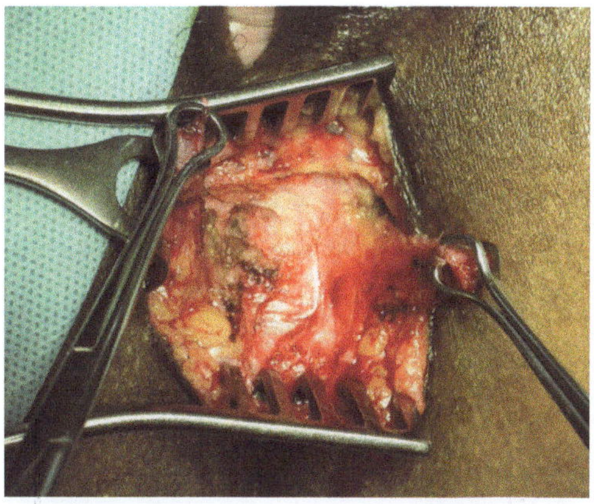

Fig. 70e. The division of the external anal sphincter

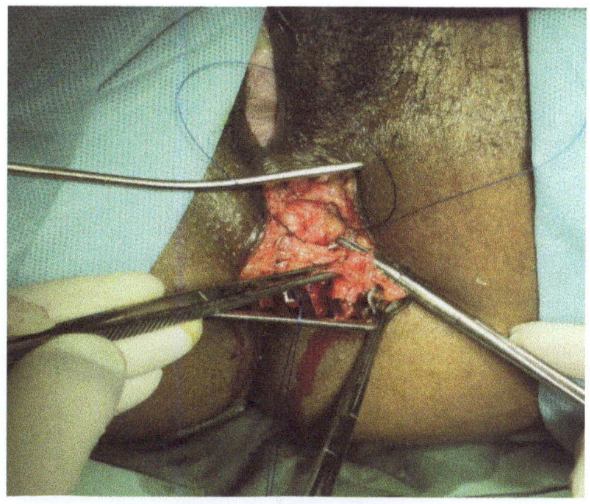

Fig. 70f. The overlapping sphincteroplasty

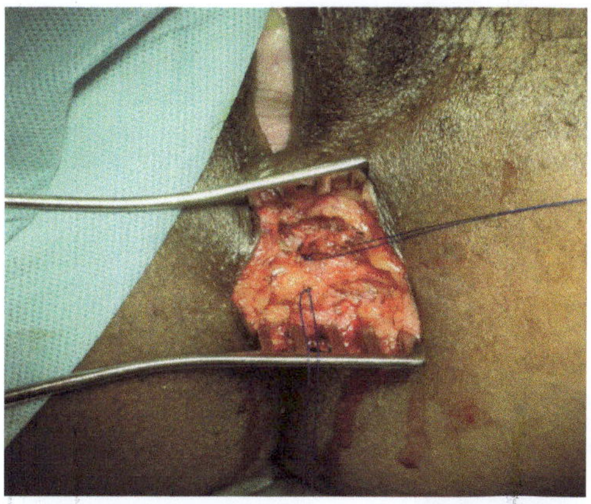

Fig. 70g. The completed repair

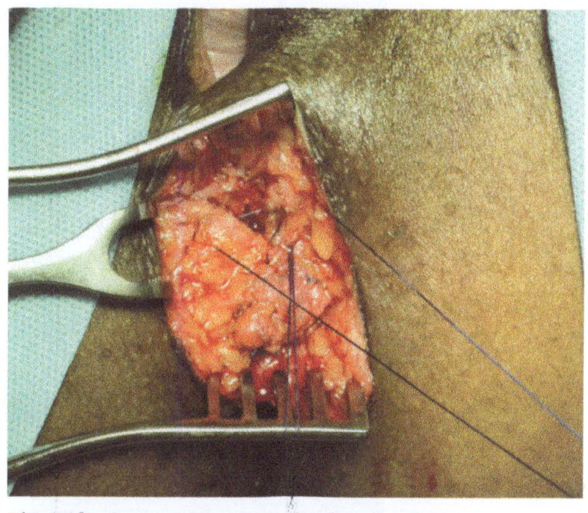

Fig. 70h. Concomitant anterior levatorplasty

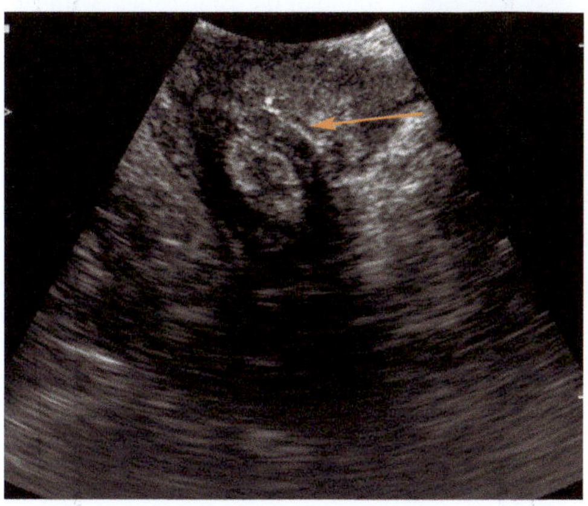

Fig. 70i. Transperineal ultrasound at one week. This shows the suture material in the overlapping external anal sphincteroplasty (*arrow*) and confirms that the rostral extent of the repair is adequate by tilting of the axial transducer against the anterior aspect of the anus

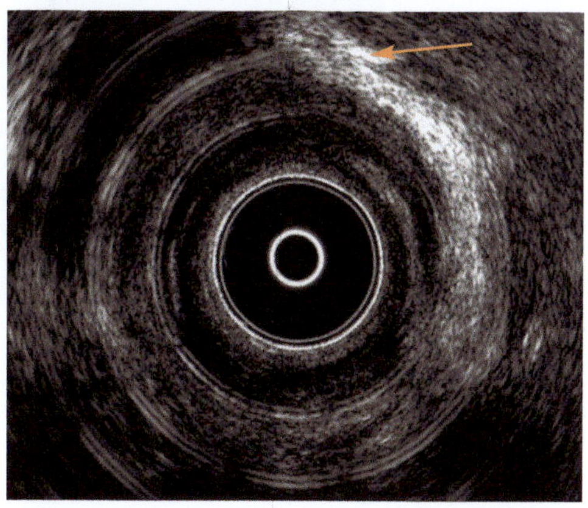

Fig. 70l. The appearances match that normally seen with endoanal ultrasound at 2 months following the sphincteroplasty (*arrow*)

Anal Fistula

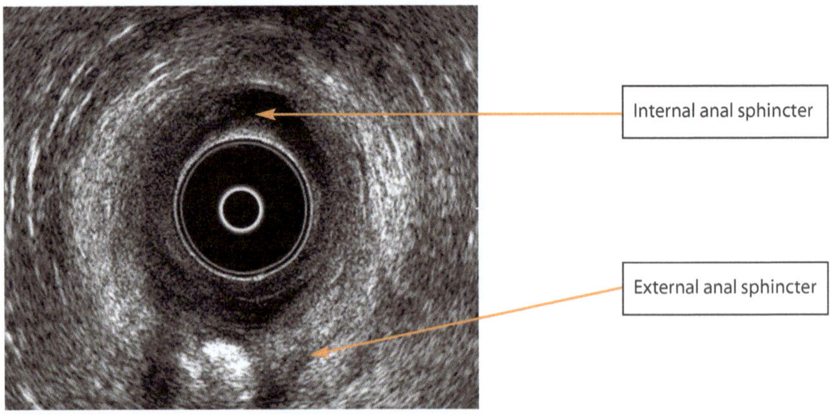

Fig. 71a. A 38 year-old Haitian man presented to our coloproctologic unit after a third operation for a fistula-in-ano. The figure shows the endoanal ultrasound with enhancement by hydrogen peroxide of the fistula extending to the level of the puborectalis. There is evidence of internal anal sphincter thinning at the point of fistula entry (7 o'clock position)

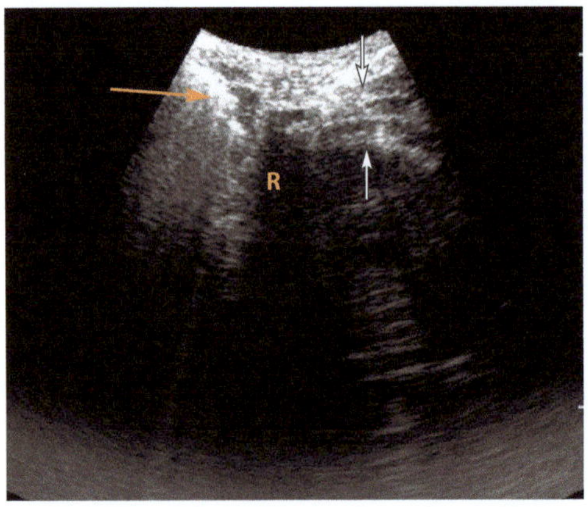

Fig. 71b. A sagittal transperineal ultrasound of the same patient with evidence of a secondary intersphincteric track (*arrows*) seen extending along the side of the anal canal. This extended to the level of the puborectalis.In the sagittal transperineal ultrasound, the anal canal is best identified by observing the parallel hypoechoic lines of the internal anal sphincter in profile (*white arrowheads*). *R*=the air-filled rectum

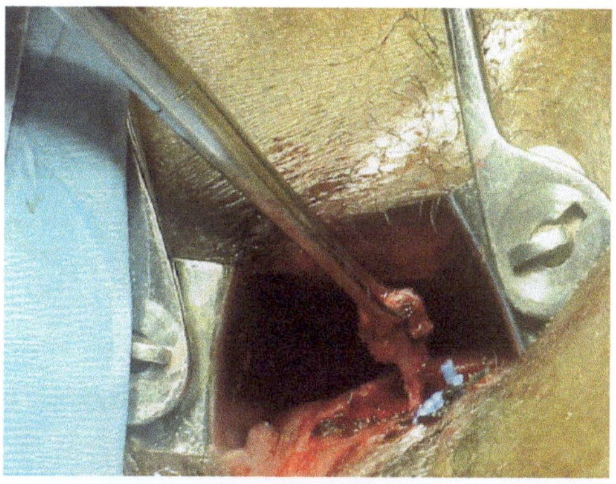

Fig. 71c. This patient was initially treated with a soft latex draining seton and at 10 weeks time after this procedure was repaired with a mucosal advancement anoplasty. This shows dissection of the fistula and seton

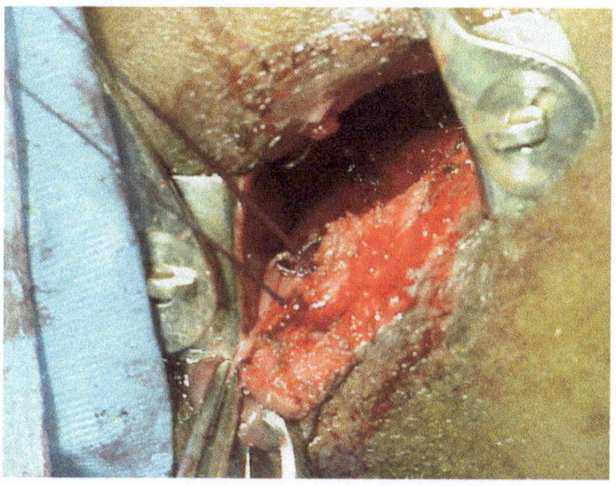

Fig. 71d. Repair of the internal anal sphincter rather than preliminary internal anal sphincterotomy prior to mucosal advancement

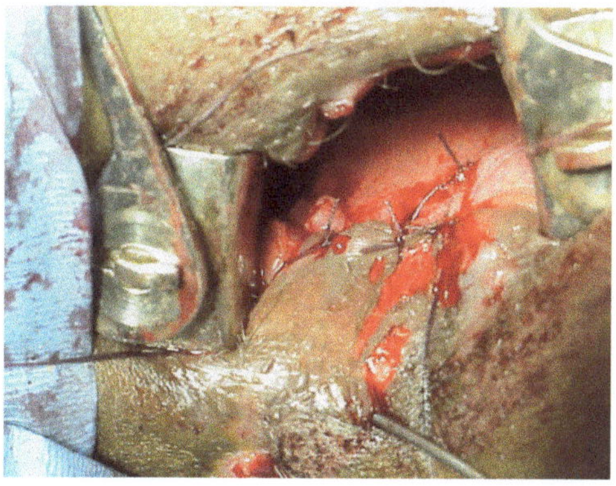

Fig. 71e. The mucosal advancement appearance. The probe demonstrates the site of the intersphincteric secondary track which was laied open

Recto-Vaginal Fistula

Transperineal sonography is particularly adept at demonstrating recto- and anovaginal fistulae which lie beyond the focal distance of endoluminal ultrasound or MR probes [15]. The fistula track can be traced with hydrogen peroxide enhancement.

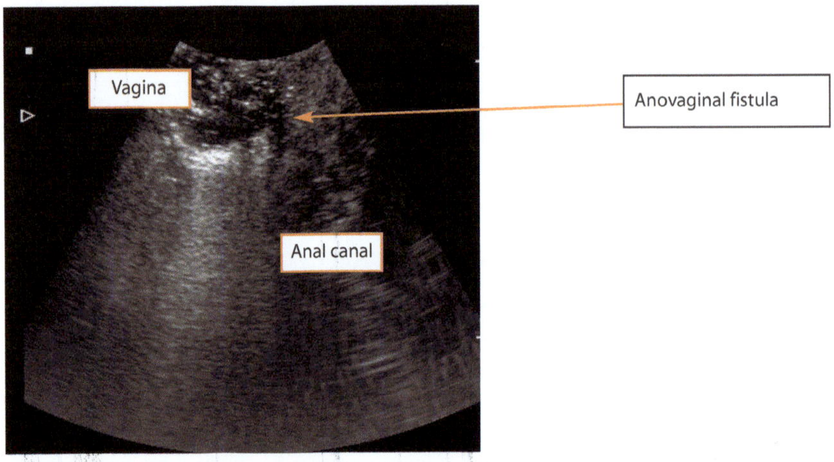

Fig. 72a. The vagina has been instilled with 50 mL of acoustic gel with a branched anovaginal fistula evident on sagittal scanning (*arrow*)

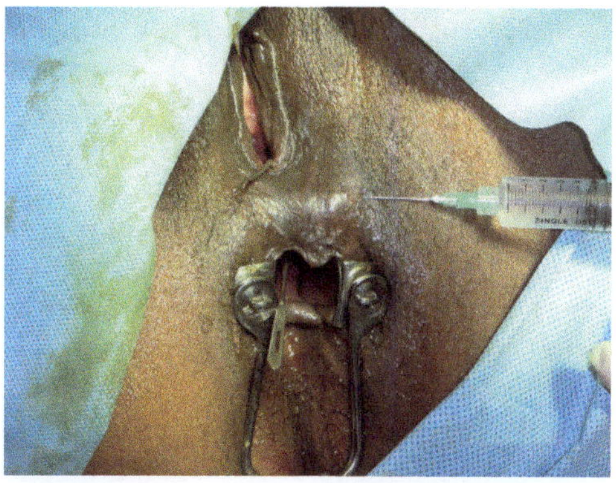

Fig. 72b. Operative slide of the anovaginal fistula with a Lockhart-Mummery probe

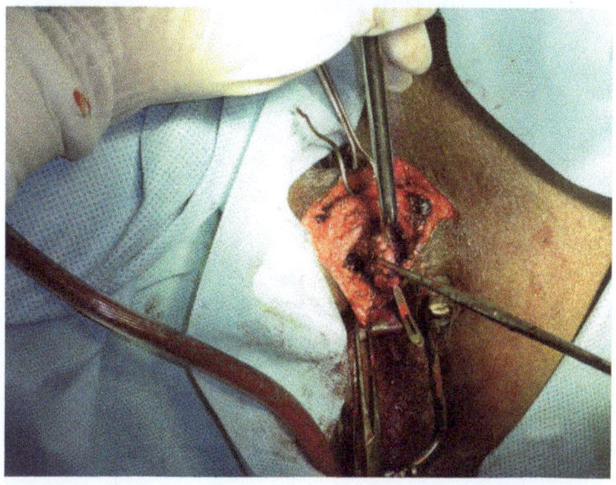

Fig. 72c. Fistula excision with rerouting after initial vaginal and endoanal mucosal repair

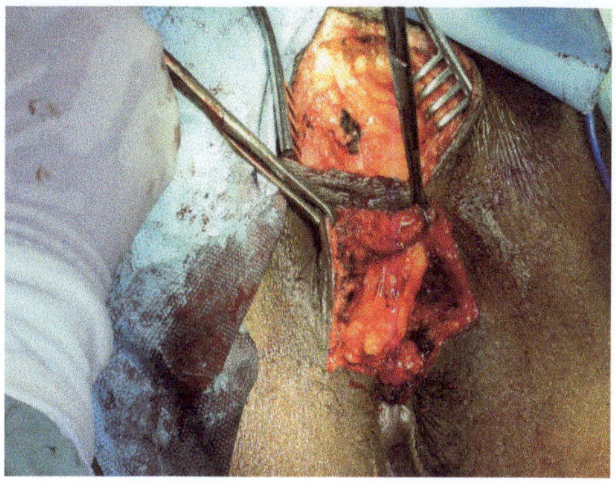

Fig. 72d. Interposition of bulbospongiosus Martius graft

Transperineal Ultrasound in Evacuatory Dysfunction

Transperineal sonography is used in dynamic mode with simulated evacuation of intrarectal acoustic gel in those patients presenting with the problem of evacuatory difficulty. Conditions such as rectoanal intussusception, descending perineum syndrome, rectal mucosal (and full-thickness) prolapse and enterocele may be diagnosed although there is a substantial learning curve of interpretation. In order to diagnose enterocele or peritoneocele it is useful for the patient to ingest 100mL of Gastrografin where peristaltic loops of small bowel are evident in the region of the rectovaginal septum. Peritoneocele is defined as widening of the rectovaginal septum without visible peristaltic loops being evident with both conditions being diagnosed more often in the post-hysterectomy patient where culdosuspension (sacrocolpopexy) or peritoneal cul-de-sac obliteration are not routinely performed.

Rectoanal Intussusception

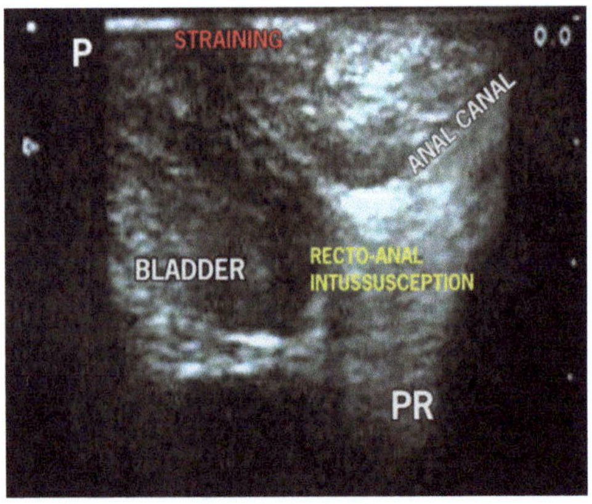

Fig. 73. The intussusception is evident as a bright echogenic intra-anal buffer during simulated defecation. *PR*=puborectalis; *P*=pubis. (Figure is provided courtesy of Dr. L. Brusciano, Italy)

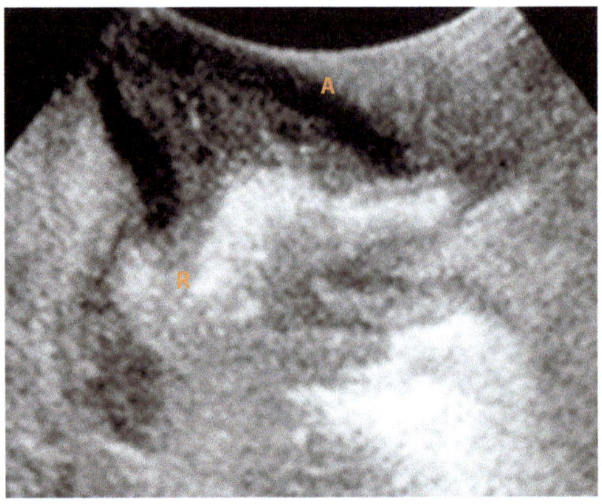

Fig. 74. Rectal intussusception buffer. *R*=rectum; *A*=anal canal. (Figure is provided courtesy of Dr. M. Beer-Gabel, Israel)

Enterocele

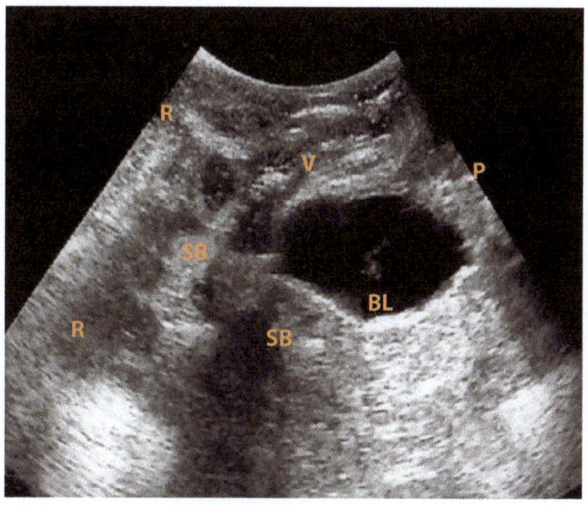

Fig. 75. The small bowel (*SB*) loops are evident in the territory of the recto-vaginal septum. *R*=rectum; *V*=vagina; *BL*=bladder; *P*=pubis. (Courtesy of Dr. M. Beer-Gabel)

Peritoneocele

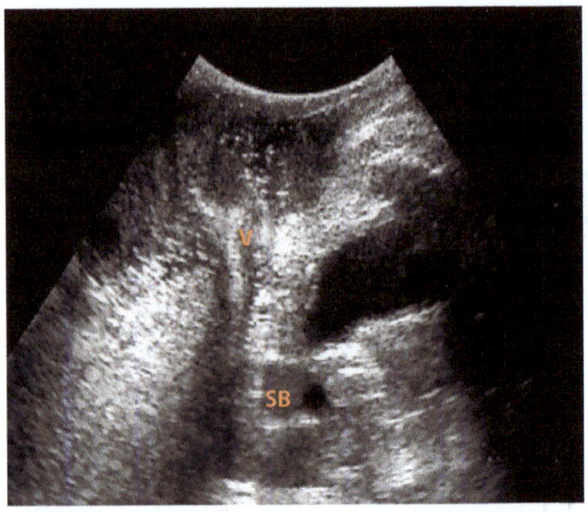

Fig. 76a. In this case, the rectogenital septum is widened. Although the small bowel is evident there is no entry or descent into the septal territory, consistent with the radiologic diagnosis of a peritoneocele. *V*=vagina; *SB*=small bowel (Courtesy of Dr. M. Beer-Gabel)

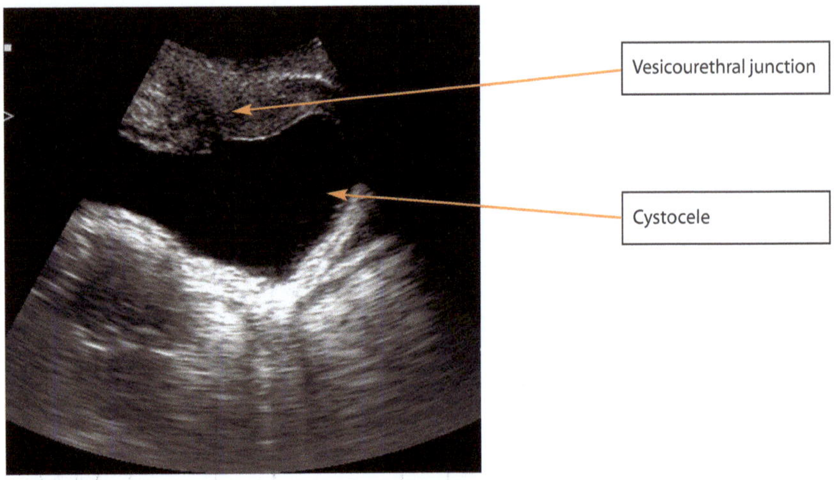

Fig. 76b. This patient also had a cystocele which was well demonstrated in the anterior sweep of the transperineal probe. Most patients presenting with evacuatory difficulty have multicompartment disease which is advantageously shown using transperineal sonography. The vesicourethral junction is well demonstrated

Rectal Prolapse

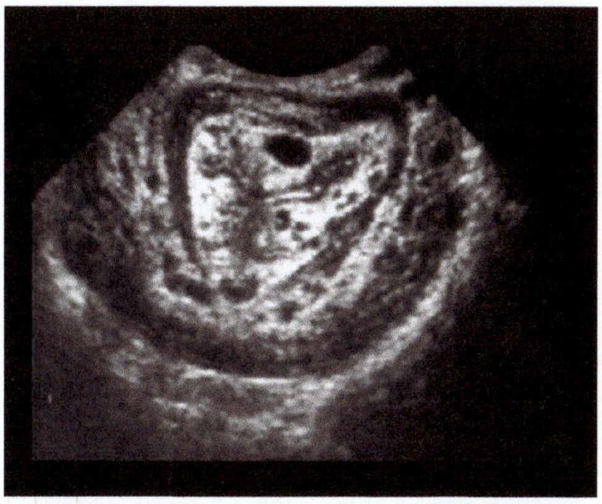

Fig. 77. Transperineal ultrasound shows the intact mucosa and Duplex scanning confirms blood flow in both hemorrhoidal disease and circumferential rectal internal mucosal prolapse (RIMP). This figure is consistent with the endoscopic diagnosis of RIMP during simulated forcible straining

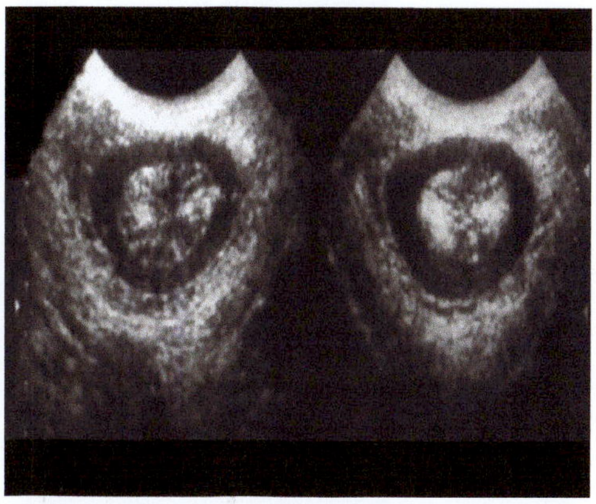

Fig. 78. The figures are the appearance at rest. (Figure courtesy of Dr. M. Beer-Gabel)

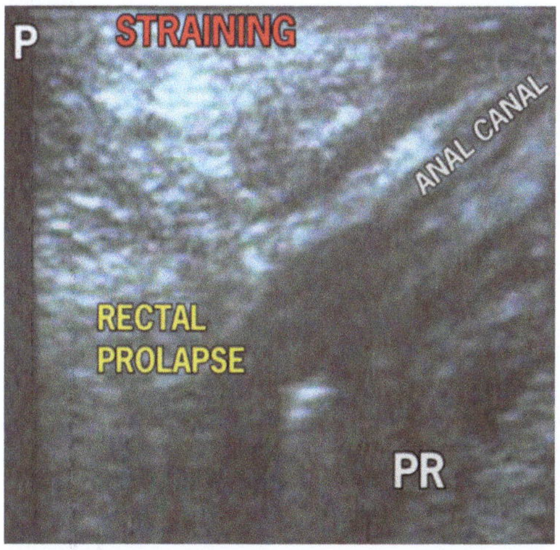

Fig. 79. Sagittal transperineal sonogram of a patient with RIMP showing an intra-anal endoluminal hyperechoic 'mass' during forcible straining commencing at the level of the puborectalis sling (*PR*). (Figure courtesy of Dr. L. Brusciano)

Rectocele

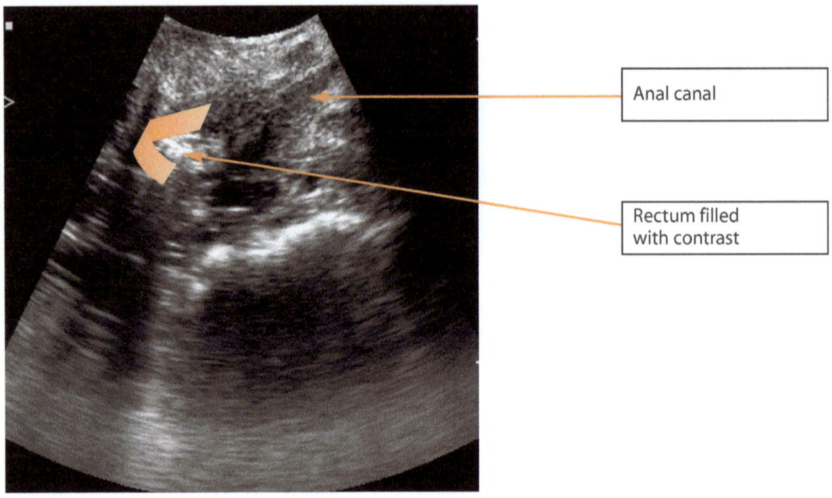

Fig. 80a. Sagittal transperineal ultrasound is most useful in confirming the clinical impression of a rectocele. Simulated defecation may also provide an estimate of the emptying capacity where rectocele depth as measured using transperineal sonography correlates well with that obtained on defecography. The rectocele is outlined and in dynamic real-time mode failed to empty

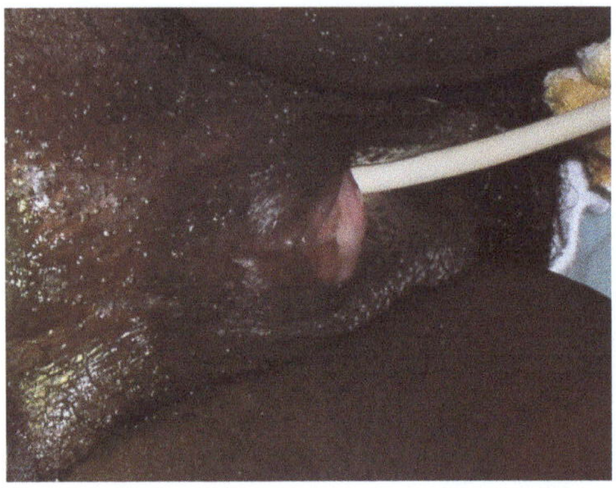

Fig. 80b. Operative slide of the rectocele with the patient in the left lateral position. The anus is posteriorly located

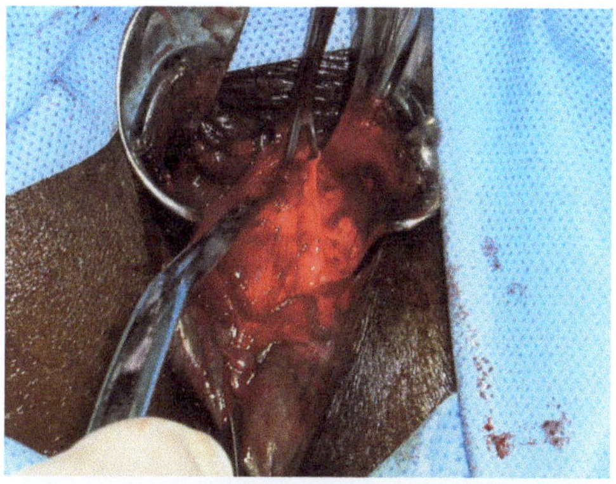

Fig. 80c. Commencement of the rectal mucosectomy. The patient is in the prone position

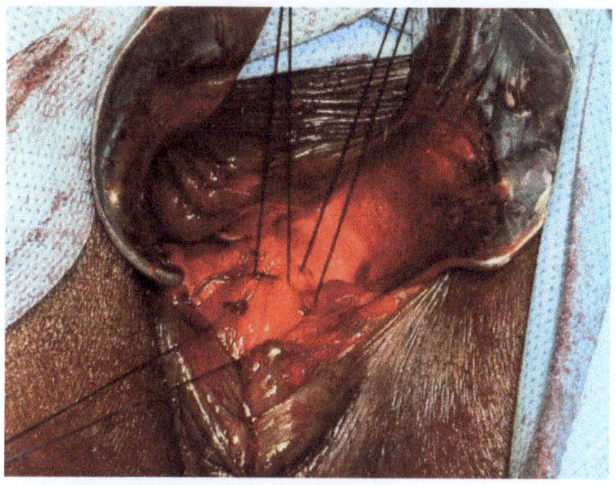

Fig. 80d. Interrupted repair of the primary defect in the rectogenital septum with vaginal protection

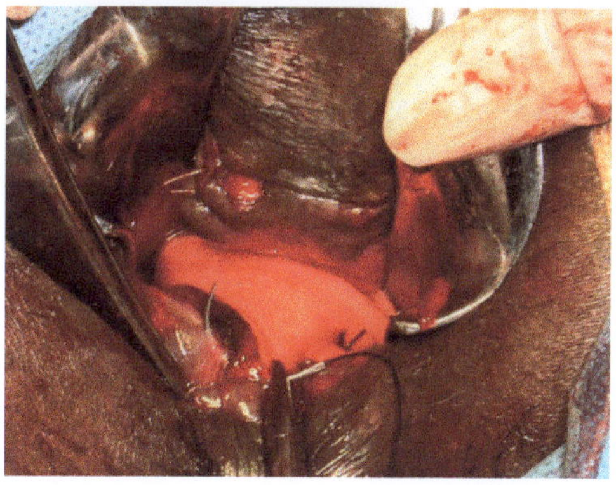

Fig. 80e. Mucosal closure after excision of redundant rectal mucosa

Evacuatory Block Due to Extra-Rectal Mass

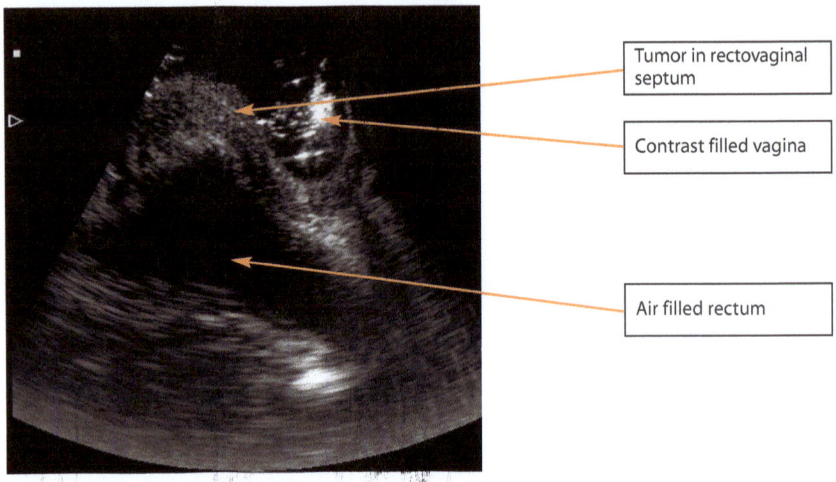

Fig. 81. In this case evacuatory difficulty was caused by a benign mesenchymal tumour originating in the recto-vaginal septum (*arrow*) which was shown on sagittal transperineal sonography. The vagina is filled with acoustic contrast. The dumb-bell tumour was removed by a combined endorectal/transperineal approach

Familial Hypertrophic Internal Sphincter

This condition has only recently been described where there is a strong family history of proctalgia accompanied by marked thickening of the hypoechoic internal anal sphincter either on endoanal or transperineal ultrasonography [16]. The condition sometimes responds to more extended internal anal sphincter myomectomy with the resected specimen showing intracytoplasmic PAS-positive inclusion bodies with specific ultrastructural inclusions on electron microscopy which are suggestive of an isolated polyglucosan storage disorder [17].

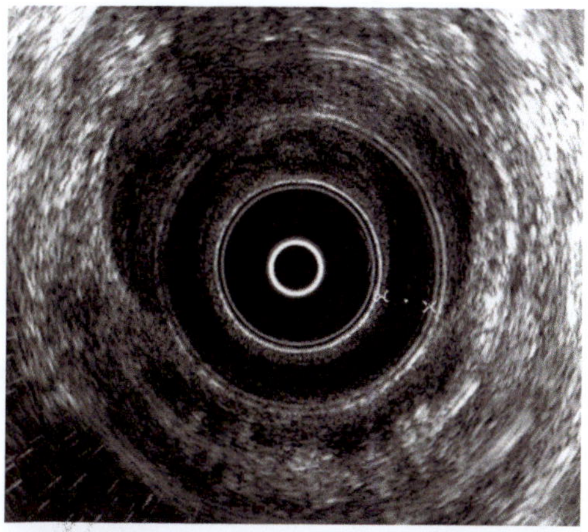

Fig. 82a. Endoanal ultrasound of a patient with internal anal sphincter myopathy who presented with a 40 year history of proctalgia which had recently been resistant to topical glyceryl trinitrate and diltiazem therapy. The diameter of the hypoechoic internal anal sphincter (marked between crosses) is 5.5 mm (normal <2 mm)

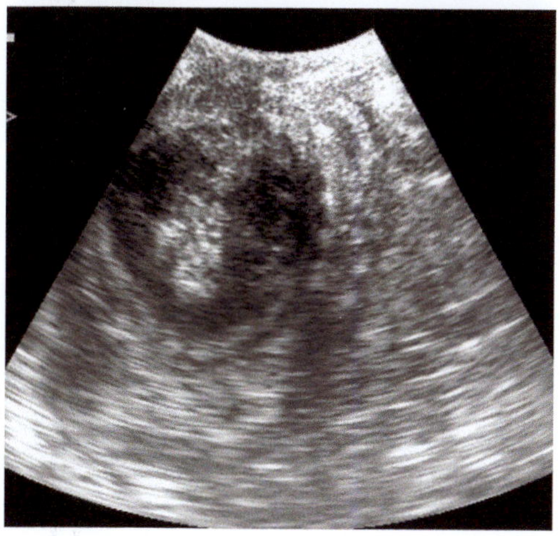

Fig. 82b. Transperineal sonogram of the same case. The maximal diameter of the internal anal sphincter recorded was 9 mm

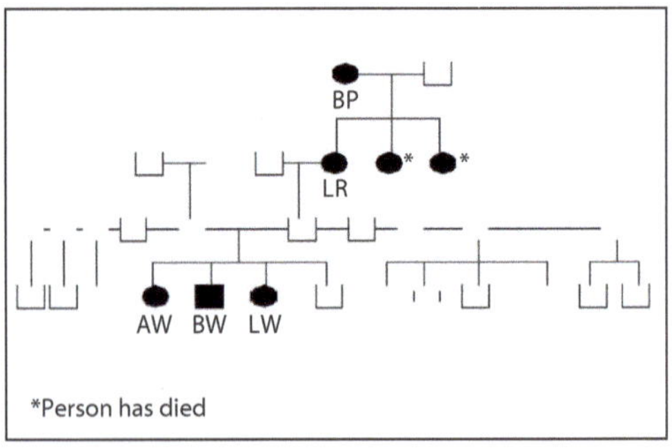

Fig. 82c. Family tree of the index case (*AW*). Shaded cases are symptomatic

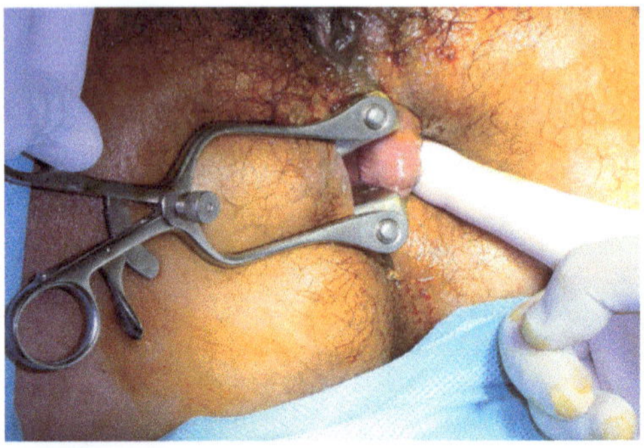

Fig. 82d. Operative appearance of grossly thickened internal anal sphincter

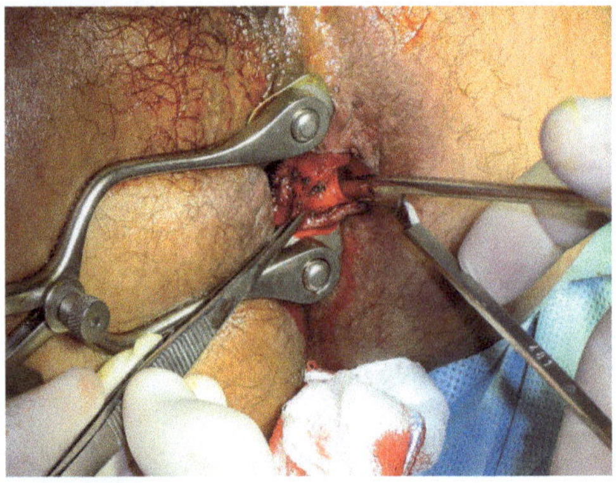

Fig. 82e. A mucosal flap was created to perform the internal anal sphincter myectomy. The grossly thickened internal anal sphincter is shown supported by some Metzenbaum scissors

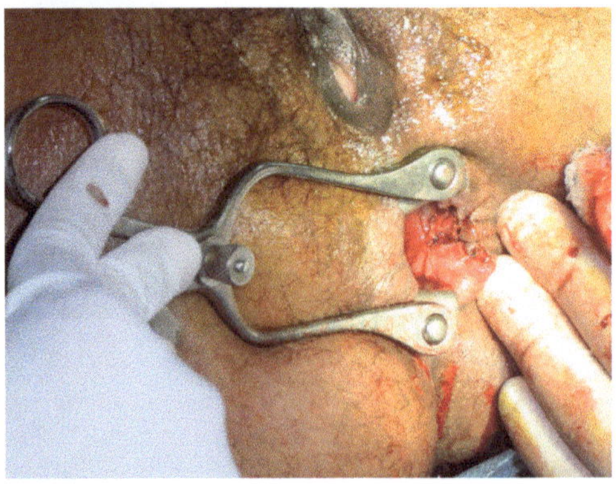

Fig. 82f. The mucosal flap was closed following sphincter excision

Imperforate Anus

Congenital anorectal anomalies are ideally suited to assessment with transperineal ultrasound, which has the capacity of demonstrating the presence or absence of components of the levator floor, low anourinary fistulae and the adequacy of both the internal and external anal sphincters. Low anovestibular fistulae can also be well shown.

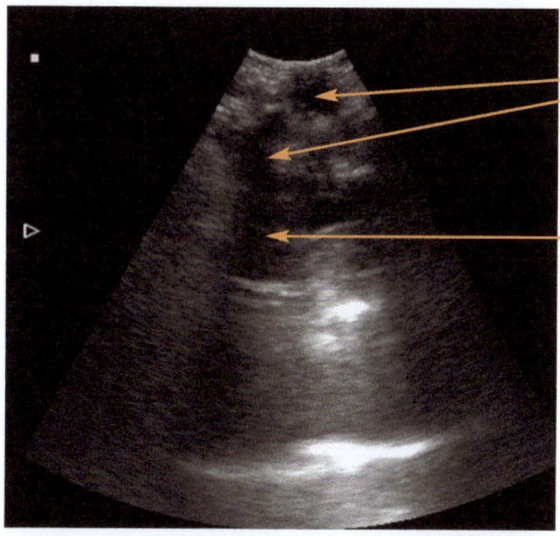

Fig. 83a. Axial transperineal sonogram showing air in the low anovestibular fistula of a one-month old baby girl. The hypoechoic internal anal sphincter is well formed

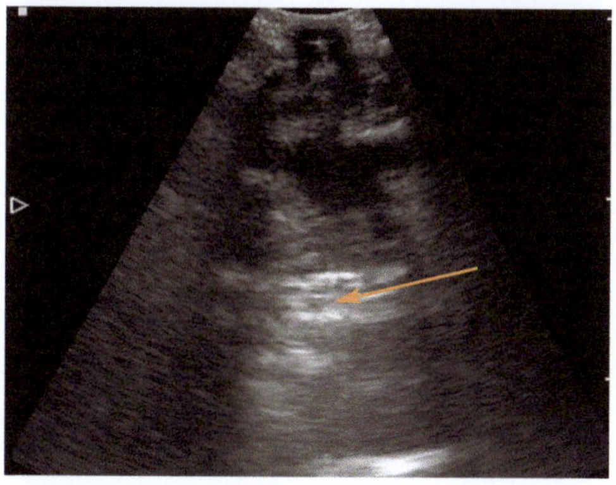

Fig. 83b. Axial sonography shows the formed hyperechoic external anal sphincter (*arrow*)

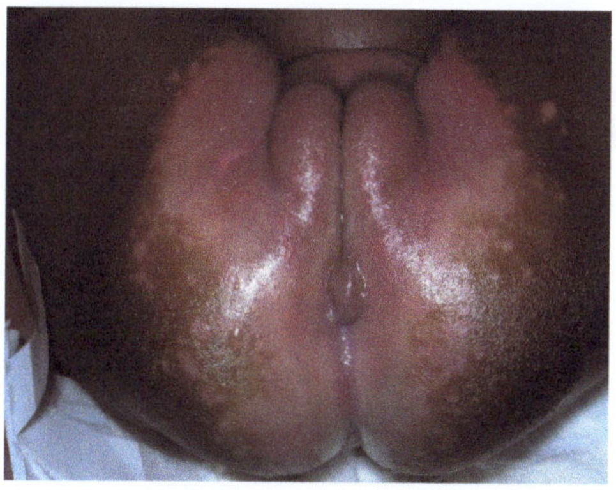

Fig. 83c. Preoperative appearance of the vestibular anus with an anovestibular fistula in a one-month old baby girl

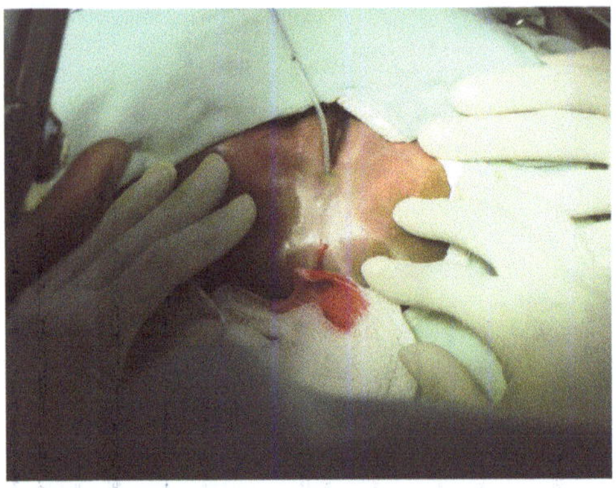

Fig. 83d. Vestibular anus is cannulated with a feeding tube

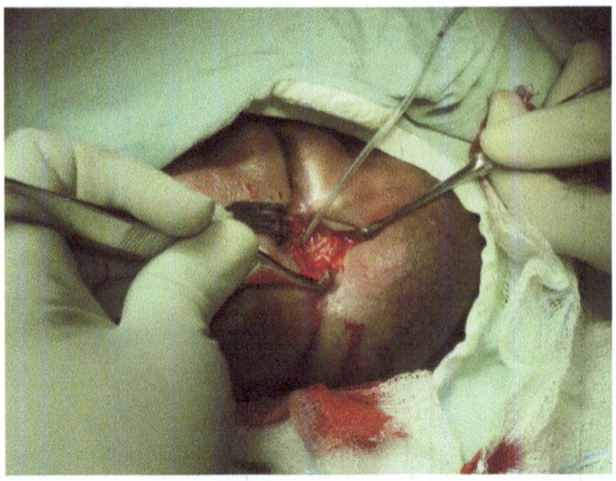

Fig. 83e. Operative picture of the commencement of the cutback anoplasty

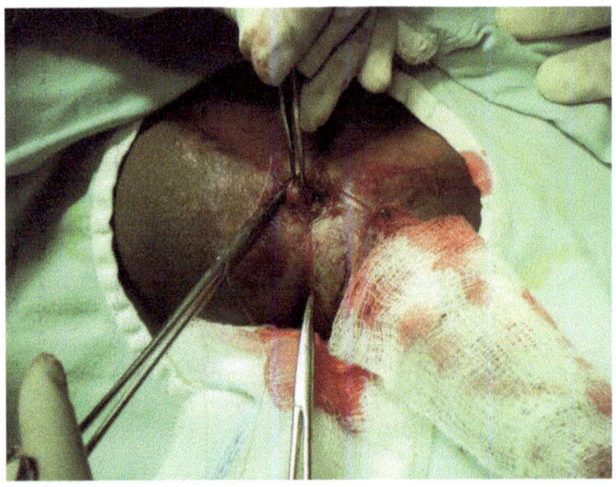

Fig. 83f. Formation of the anoplasty

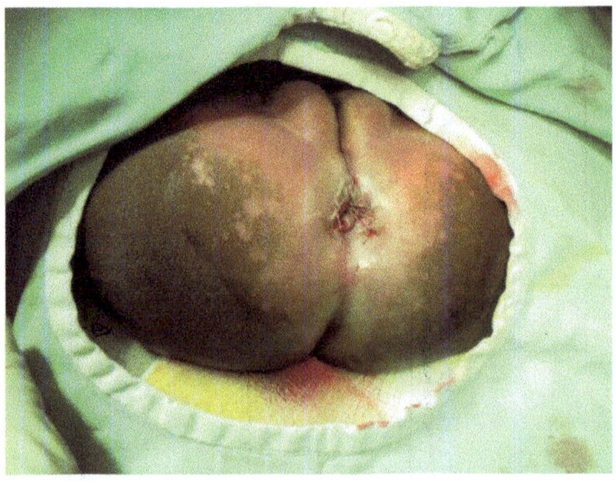

Fig. 83g. Completion anoplasty result

Operative photographs (Figs. 83d-g) of this child are courtesy of Dr. S. Jackman and Dr. A. Peters, Queen Elizabeth Hospital, Barbados.

References

1. Koebl H, Bernaschek G, Dentinger J (1990) Assessment of female urinary incontinence by introital sonography. J Clin Ultrasound 18:370-374
2. Schaer GN, Koechli OR, Scheussler B, Haller U (1995) Perineal ultrasound for evaluating the bladder neck in urinary stress incontinence. Obstet Gynecol 85:220-224
3. Kleinubing H Jr, Janini JF, Malafaia O, Brenner S, Pinho M (2000) Transperineal ultrasonography: new method to image the anorectal region. Dis Colon Rectum 43:1572-1574
4. Piloni V (2001) Dynamic imaging of the pelvic floor with transperineal sonography. Tech Coloproctol 5:103-105
5. Beer-Gabel M, Teshler M, Barzilai N, Lurie Y, Malnick S, Bass D, Zbar A (2002) Dynamic transperineal ultrasound in the diagnosis of pelvic floor disorders: pilot study. Dis Colon Rectum 45:239-248
6. Beer-Gabel M, Teshler M, Schechtman E, Zbar AP (2004) Dynamic transperineal ultrasound versus defecography in patients with evacuatory difficulty: a pilot study. Int J Colorectal Dis 19:60-67
7. Cruiskshank SH (1991) Sacrospinous fixation- should this be performed at the time of vaginal hysterectomy? Am J Obstet Gynecol 164:1072-1076
8. Backer MH (1992) Success with sacrospinous suspension of the prolapsed vaginal vault. Surg Gynecol Obstet 175:419-420
9. McCall ML (1997) Posterior culdoplasty: surgical correction of enterocele during vaginal hysterectomy. A preliminary report. Obstet Gynecol 10:596-602
10. Beer-Gabel M, Zbar AP (2002) Dynamic transperineal ultrasonography (DTP-US) in patients presenting with obstructed defecation. Tech Coloproctol 6:141
11. Zbar AP, Lienemann A, Fritsch H, Beer-Gabel M, Pescatori M (2003) Rectocele: pathogenesis and surgical management. Int J Colorectal Dis 18:369-384
12. Mallouhi A, Bonatti H, Peer S, Lugger P, Conrad F, Bodner G (2004) Detection and characterization of perianal inflammatory disease. Accuracy of transperineal combined gray scale and color Doppler sonography. J Ultrasound Med 23:19-27
13. Wedemeyer J, Kirchhoff T, Sellge G, Bachmann O, Lotz J, Galanski M, Manns MP, Gebel MJ, Bleck JS (2004) Transcutaneous perianal sonography: a sensitive method for the detection of perianal inflammatory lesions in Crohn's disease. World J Gastroenterol 10:2859-2863
14. Kim I-O, Han TI, Kim WS, Yeon KM (2000) Transperineal ultrasonography in imperforate anus: identification of the internal fistula. J Ultrasound Med 19:211-216
15. Laurence FY, Birnbaum EH, Read TE, Kodner IJ, Fleshman JW (1999) Use of endoanal ultrasound in patients with rectovaginal fistulas. Dis Colon Rectum 42:1057-1064
16. Kamm MA, Hoyle CH, Burleigh DE, Law PJ, Swash M, Martin JE, Nicholls RJ, Northover JM (1991) Hereditary internal anal sphincter myopathy causing proctalgia fugax and constipation. A newly defined condition. Gastroenterology 100:805-810
17. Thompson AJ, Swash M, Cox`EL, Ingram DJ, Gray A, Schwartz NS (1988) Polysaccharide storage myopathy. Muscle Nerve 11:349-355

Conclusions

This atlas combines a surgical knowledge of anal sonography with an operative decision-making approach for specific benign proctologic disorders as referred to a tertiary coloproctological practice. The advantages and disadvantages of two- and three-dimensional, transvaginal and transperineal sonography are outlined with practical examples displaying the specific information obtained from each modality for successful surgical outcomes in complex perirectal sepsis, fecal incontinence, functional evacuation disorders and in a range of miscellaneous proctological disorders, including persistent proctalgia and congenital anorectal anomalies and their aftermath. With each modality the clinician should realize that the appropriate imaging may be utilized to answer different but specific questions which aid in management, and that these techniques may be more complementary than competitive where the benefits of one modality may provide useful information not rendered by the other techniques. The surgeon must liaise closely with the radiologist in order to obtain the most useful understanding of the problem and to be able to interpret an overall three-dimensional comprehension of the condition based on relevant preoperative imaging. It is axiomatic to state that surgeons do not operate solely on images and that these images obtained with different modalities must be correlated with the clinical impression for optimal results. The nature of training and accreditation of anal ultrasonography (in all its forms) remains to be firmly established but it is reasonable to expect that this area will be formalized in the coming years.

MIX
Papier aus verantwortungsvollen Quellen
Paper from responsible sources
FSC® C105338

If you have any concerns about our products,
you can contact us on
ProductSafety@springernature.com

In case Publisher is established outside the EU,
the EU authorized representative is:
Springer Nature Customer Service Center GmbH
Europaplatz 3, 69115 Heidelberg, Germany

Printed by Libri Plureos GmbH
in Hamburg, Germany